Psychology of Rehabilitation

Edited by **Brian Bolton, Ph.D.**, Associate Professor of Rehabilitation and Adjunct Associate Professor of Psychology, University of Arkansas

Deafness as a devastating handicap manifested by severe linguistic retardation and impaired communication skills is the major theme of the nine chapters in this volume. The book outlines for practitioners in the helping professions the psychological circumstances of deaf persons, and it describes the principles, procedures, and techniques proven valuable in the rehabilitation of deaf clients.

Each chapter summarizes one particular area of life functioning of deaf persons. The first chapter presents an overview of the main topics; the next six chapters focus on specific areas of development and functioning: communicative, intellectual, personality, vocational, academic, and psychiatric aspects of deafness. Two concluding chapters outline principles of program development in early education and rehabilitation.

Psychology of Deafness for Rehabilitation Counselors summarizes knowledge acquired by its distinguished authors — all acknowledged authorities in psychology, deafness, and education — during many years of teaching, counseling, and studying deaf people. It provides a basic, comprehensive, and authoritative text and reference for rehabilitation counselors, social workers, educators, and other social science practitioners. It is recommended as a primary textbook for in-service training and for preparatory courses in psychology of deafness, introduction to deafness, and counseling with deaf persons. It is also a valuable collateral reference for professionals investigating psychological aspects of disability and rehabilitation.

Psychology of Deafness for Rehabilitation Counselors

Psychology
of Deafness
for
Rehabilitation
Counselors

Edited by
Brian Bolton, Ph.D.

**Arkansas Rehabilitation Research
and Training Center
University of Arkansas**

University Park Press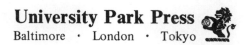
Baltimore · London · Tokyo

UNIVERSITY PARK PRESS
International Publishers in Science and Medicine
Chamber of Commerce Building
Baltimore, Maryland 21202

Typeset by The Composing Room of Michigan, Inc.

Manufactured in the United States of America by Universal Lithographers, Inc., and The Maple Press Co.

Library of Congress Cataloging in Publication Data
Main entry under title:

Psychology of deafness for rehabilitation counselors.

Includes index.
  1. Deafness—Psychological aspects—Addresses, essays, lectures. 2. Deaf—Rehabilitation—Addresses, essays, lectures. I. Bolton, Brian F. [DNLM: 1. Deafness—Rehabilitation. 2. Counseling. HV2395 P974]
HV2395.P75   362.4'2'019   76-4857
ISBN 0-8391-0926-1

Contents

Contributors

Kenneth Z. Altshuler is Professor of Clinical Psychiatry at Columbia University's College of Physicians and Surgeons. Dr. Altshuler received his M.D. from the University of Buffalo and is a Training Analyst at Columbia University's Psychoanalytic Clinic for Training and Research, Director of Undergraduate Education at the College of Physicians and Surgeons, and the Unit Chief of New York State's special unit for the deaf. He has authored over 70 articles and books based on his extensive research in the fields of genetics, geriatrics, early total deafness, psychoanalysis, and sleep and dreams as they relate to psychiatry. His work received the Thornton Wilson Award in genetics and preventive psychiatry in 1961, the merit award of the Association for Psychoanalytic Medicine in 1963, and he was awarded an Honorary Doctorate of Science from Gallaudet College in 1972.

Brian Bolton is Associate Professor of Rehabilitation and Adjunct Associate Professor of Psychology at the University of Arkansas. He received his Ph.D. from the University of Wisconsin. Dr. Bolton authored *Introduction to Rehabilitation Research* (1974) and edited the *Handbook of Measurement and Evaluation in Rehabilitation* (1976) and is the author or co-author of numerous journal articles, research monographs, conference presentations, and reviews in rehabilitation, deafness, and psychometrics. He has received several awards for his research and is currently Associate Editor of the *Rehabilitation Counseling Bulletin.*

Harry Bornstein is Research Professor of Psychology at Gallaudet College. He received his Ph.D. from American University. Dr. Bornstein, who is a fellow of the American Psychological Association and the American Association for the Advancement of Science, is the author of more than 30 publications in the areas of psychometrics and deafness. He is also the principal author of the 45 titles in the Signed English Series for deaf children.

Harry W. Hoemann is Associate Professor of Psychology at Bowling Green State University. He received his Ph.D. from Catholic University. Dr. Hoemann's research interests center on the development of communication skills in deaf children. Together with his wife he has developed instructional materials for American Sign Language published by the National Association for the Deaf. Dr. Hoemann is the author of more than 40 publications and presentations in deafness and related areas.

Helen S. Lane is Psychologist and Consultant, Principal Emeritus at the Central Institute for the Deaf, and Professor of Education in the Department of Speech and Hearing at Washington University. She received her Ph.D. from Ohio State University and was President of the A. G. Bell Association from 1965 to 1969. Dr. Lane's distinguished career in deafness includes the publication of more than 50 articles and book chapters. She is a Fellow of the American Psychological Association and received the Silver Fawn Award in 1974 from the Boy Scouts of America for her work in the scouting program for deaf boys at the Central Institute and as a consultant for the Handbook for Deaf Scouts.

Alan Lerman is Director of Research at the Lexington School for the Deaf in New York City. He has directed a series of major research projects, spanning 12 years, specifically related to the vocational development of the deaf. He received his Ph.D. from New York University where he subsequently taught courses in the Psychology of Deafness and conducted Seminars on Research in Deafness. Dr. Lerman has directed and participated in the development of seminal programs on infant services, mental health, special learning disorders, and bilingual education for deaf children.

Kathryn R. Meadow is Associate Adjunct Professor of Sociology, Department of Psychiatry, at the University of California (San Francisco) and Research Director, Mental Health Services for the Deaf, Langley Porter Neuropsychiatric Institute. She received her Ph.D. from the University of California (Berkeley). Dr. Meadow co-authored *Sound and Sign: Childhood Deafness and Mental Health* (1973) and has published more than 40 articles, chapters, and monographs on deafness. She has served as consultant and lecturer to numerous organizations and universities and received the Daniel T. Cloud Award in 1974 for her contributions to the field of deafness.

Audrey Simmons-Martin is Director of Early Education at the Central Institute for the Deaf and Professor of Education at Washington University (St. Louis). She received her Ed.D. from Washington University. Dr. Simmons-Martin has authored some 35 articles and book chapters focused on deaf children and their parents. Dr. Simmons-Martin is a Fellow of the American Speech and Hearing Association. She has received several awards recognizing her contributions to deaf education, including the St. Louis 1970 Woman of Achievement citation.

Norman L. Tully is Professor of Counseling and Director of the Rehabilitation Counseling with the Deaf Program at Gallaudet College. He received his Ed.D. from the University of Arizona. Dr. Tully, who has extensive counseling, teaching, and administrative experience in deaf education and rehabilitation, has authored and co-authored several articles pertaining to deafness and rehabilitation.

Douglas Ullman is Assistant Professor of Psychology at Bowling Green State University. Dr. Ullman received his Ph.D. from the University of Iowa and is a clinical child psychologist and serves as a consultant in the area of mental retardation. He is the author or co-author of several articles and presentations on deafness and assessment.

James C. Woodward is Assistant Professor of English and Linguistics at Gallaudet College. He received his Ph.D. from Georgetown University. Dr. Woodward teaches undergraduate and graduate courses and conducts research at the Linguistics Research Laboratory at Gallaudet. He is the author or co-author of some two dozen publications and presentations in linguistics and deafness.

Preface

Psychologists have conducted numerous investigations designed to advance the understanding of the impact of deafness on human functioning and to develop techniques and programs for assisting deaf persons to adjust to their unique disability. Deafness, while constituting an invisible handicap to the naïve observer is, in reality, a devastating disability. The inability to hear the spoken word prevents the normal acquisition of the predominant mode of human communication—language. Thus, deafness as a handicapping condition is manifested as severe linguistic retardation and impaired communication skills. This is the major theme that runs through the nine chapters comprising this volume.

The purpose of *Psychology of Deafness for Rehabilitation Counselors* is to outline for practitioners in the helping professions the psychological circumstances of deaf persons and to describe principles, procedures, and techniques that have proven valuable in rehabilitation of deaf clients. The first chapter presents an overview of the major topics covered in the following eight chapters. Six chapters focus on specific areas of development and functioning: communicative, intellectual, personality, vocational, academic, and psychiatric aspects of deafness. Two chapters outline principles of program development in early education and rehabilitation. One conspicuous omission is a chapter on psychological evaluation of the deaf client; the interested reader is referred to Edna S. Levine's excellent chapter in the *Handbook of Measurement and Evaluation in Rehabilitation* (1976) (also published by University Park Press). Rehabilitation counselors, social workers, educators, and other social service practitioners should find *Psychology of Deafness for Rehabilitation Counselors* to be a useful introduction to the world of deafness.

Professionals who work with deaf adults in rehabilitation settings must be conversant in the language of signs and fingerspelling. The easiest way to acquire the necessary skills is through interaction with deaf persons. Local speech and hearing clinics or the Registry of Interpreters for the Deaf (RID) can provide information on sign language classes and recommend tutors. Information regarding various professional training programs is available from the Professional Rehabilitation Workers with the Adult Deaf (PRWAD).

This volume summarizes the knowledge that has been acquired during many years of experience in teaching, counseling, and studying deaf persons by the distinguished authors of the chapters. Their contributions to the field of rehabilitation are greatly appreciated. Special thanks are given to Diane Graham who assisted with the preparation of the manuscript and assembled the index for the book.

A brief cautionary remark is appropriate at this point. Our knowledge of the impact of deafness on the linguistic development, intellectual functioning, academic achievement, and personal-social adjustment of deaf persons, while substantial, is far from complete. It follows, then, that considerable differences of opinion exist regarding optimal educational programs for deaf children and, to a lesser extent, rehabilitation techniques appropriate for deaf young adults. Thus, the diversity in orientation which characterizes the chapters of this book simply reflects the current state of knowledge. The reader should recognize the different philosophies or "schools of thought" for what they are: conclusions that the authors have reached based on their interpretations of incomplete evidence pertaining to a highly complex subject.

1 | Introduction and Overview

BRIAN BOLTON

The purpose of this first chapter is to provide the reader with a global survey of the characteristics of young deaf rehabilitation clients. Each of the topics which is overviewed in this chapter is considered in greater depth in subsequent chapters. Although the focus is on young adults, most of the conclusions apply with equal accuracy to older deaf persons. By extending optimal service to young adults, rehabilitation workers hope to reduce the number of maladjusted deaf adults in future decades.

MAGNITUDE OF PROBLEM

More than 3,000 youth aged 16–19 years leave schools and classes for the deaf annually. Roughly 15% enter Gallaudet College, the National Technical Institute for the Deaf, or other college-level programs. Several hundred enroll in technical-vocational schools and community colleges which provide special arrangements for deaf students. An unknown number begin apprenticeships or on-the-job training programs. Many enter the job market at the clerical, semiskilled, and unskilled levels. Others become unemployed or enter intensive rehabilitation programs. Theoretically, all deaf youth are eligible for rehabilitation services sponsored by the state-

Preparation of *Psychology of Deafness for Rehabilitation Counselors* was supported in part by Rehabilitation Services Administration Grant 16-P-56812 to the Arkansas Rehabilitation Research and Training Center.

1

federal vocational rehabilitation program, and a substantial proportion do become clients sooner or later.

NEED FOR REHABILITATION SERVICES

It is doubtful whether the current programs and those which are anticipated during the next 5 years will prove adequate to meet the needs of the deaf community. The proportion of the United States population who are deaf has been relatively constant for the last 100 years. Since the population has been increasing at an accelerating rate, so has the number of deaf persons. Furthermore, because of advances in medical science, the proportion of children deafened postlingually (after the age of 4 years) has decreased markedly. More than 95% of deaf children of primary school age today were either born deaf or were deafened before the age of 2 years (90% were born deaf). Thus, in absolute magnitude, the number of deaf persons is increasing, and the educational problems which they present are increasing in level of difficulty. Until some breakthroughs in the education of deaf children are realized, there will be an increasing need for rehabilitation services for deaf young adults.

CHARACTERISTICS OF DEAF YOUNG ADULTS

Sufficient information is available to construct a composite picture of the deaf young adult in the United States. It is important to remember that what follows reflects the average; considerable variability exists within this subpopulation.

Language Development and Communication Skills

Most deaf persons learn to communicate reasonably well using manual sign language (including fingerspelling), but their formal language skills, as exemplified by reading comprehension and written communication, are very poor. The most recent comprehensive study indicates that the average deaf 16-year-old person has attained the reading skills of the average hearing fourth grader (Office of Demographic Studies, 1972b). Fewer than 10% read at or beyond the seventh grade level. At least one-third of deaf youth are functionally illiterate.

Educational Achievement

Achievement in other areas is only slightly better, e.g., the median grade equivalent in spelling and arithmetic computation for deaf 16-year-olds is sixth grade. In general, rote skills are taught and mastered somewhat more easily than problem-solving or synthetic skills, but substantial retardation is still evident. A liberal estimate of the proportion of deaf persons who ever attain a median achievement level of twelfth grade would be 1%.

Intellectual Functioning

The cognitive skills of deaf children and youth have been extensively investigated. The question of singular importance concerns the impact of auditory deprivation on intellectual development and functioning. Since deafness is almost synonymous with linguistic retardation, the question reduces to the relationship between linguistic facility and cognitive development. A large number of investigations conducted during the past 50 years has conclusively demonstrated that intellectual development and functioning are not dependent on language skills and that deaf persons possess normal intelligence. This is a very important conclusion because it implies that deaf persons have the potential to achieve to the same degree as hearing persons.

Personality Development and Social Functioning

It has been hypothesized that early childhood deafness and the subsequent retarded language development would produce impairments in personality development. However, the research evidence does not support the hypothesis of personality malformation or dysfunction as a result of deafness, although many deaf young adults do exhibit patterns of behavior reflecting retarded emotional development and immature social functioning. This delayed personal-social development can be attributed to growing up in a sheltered, overprotective environment, and not to deafness per se.

Vocational Development

A recent investigation of the vocational development of deaf youth documented their vocational immaturity in comparison to hearing peers (Lerman and Guilfoyle, 1970). In this study, deaf adolescents expressed preferences for occupations at semiskilled and unskilled levels, their vocational interests were less crystallized, and they possessed less vocational information than hearing adolescents. Survey studies have found deaf workers to be generally satisfied and rated as satisfactory employees in their semiskilled and unskilled jobs. Despite the fact that deaf youth have a restricted view of the world of work and often receive inadequate vocational preparation, a substantial proportion eventually do make an acceptable, if minimal, vocational adjustment.

THREE MYTHS ABOUT DEAFNESS

The following paragraphs summarize three widely held beliefs about deaf persons which act to further complicate the already difficult problems confronting educators and rehabilitators.

Myth of Lipreading

The typical layman believes that deaf persons communicate by lipreading (more appropriately termed speechreading). This false notion is maintained by the popular media and the oral educational establishment. The truth of the matter is that very few deaf persons can speechread with any degree of proficiency. In fact, the indistinguishability of many visible speech elements makes the task almost impossible. Research studies indicate that hearing persons are better speechreaders than most deaf persons who have undergone several years of training. Their superior knowledge of the structure of language enables hearing persons to guess many of the otherwise indistinguishable words from the context in which they occur.

Myth of Concrete Thinking

Until recently, psychologists believed that deaf persons were lacking in abstract thinking capacity and that they could function normally only if restricted to concrete activities. The source of the misunderstanding that occurred was semantic: concreteness referred to deaf subjects' difficulty in dealing with language-dependent concepts. When intelligence tests and other assessment procedures which relied on verbal presentation or language tasks were administered to deaf persons, they performed very poorly. Their language deficiency was being measured and not an inability to deal with abstract concepts. Deaf persons do possess the intellectual capacity to solve abstract problems that do not require linguistic mediation.

Myth of Compensation

Another popular, yet fallacious, belief is that disabled persons develop compensatory abilities, e.g., deaf persons possess superior visual memory ability. The available evidence generally does not support this appealing notion (Schiff and Thayer, 1974). Deaf persons may utilize their abilities differently than hearing persons to perform the same tasks, however. In fact, this would represent a normal adjustment to disability. (This type of adjustment does not necessarily support the "organismic shift hypothesis" which is discussed in the next section, although it could be the consequence of the hypothesized phenomenon.) The myth of compensation has great appeal because it is consistent with a broader belief in universal equality and justice. The above discussion does not apply to compensation as a *motivational* concept; many disabled persons do expend exceptional amounts of energy to overcome their handicaps.

PSYCHOLOGY OF DEAFNESS

This section presents a brief summary of psychological knowledge of the effects of deafness in the following areas: language, communication skills, and intelligence; personality development and social adjustment; and abilities, interests, and attitudes.

Language, Communication Skills, and Intelligence

Language and Communication The normal nondeaf child learns the language of the society into which he is born by hearing it. When auditory input is greatly reduced, language development in the child is effectively curtailed. Language refers to the verbal-graphic symbol system that is taken for granted by most people because it seems to occur naturally. In fact, language is man's greatest achievement and his unique defining characteristic. Language is the foundation upon which our vastly complex civilization is built. Culture is transmitted through the medium of language. Language is a tool which enables man to think abstractly, i.e., to construct and manipulate mental representations to solve problems. However, language is *not* the only basis for abstraction.

Communication refers to various signaling systems which exist or develop among animals, including man. The communication systems of most animals are innately determined and serve the sole function of continuing the survival of the species. (One theoretical position regarding language acquisition in man maintains that linguistic capacity is innate, too.) Thus, communication includes a much larger range of behaviors than language; however, language provides one (highly elaborate) procedure for communication among men.

The distinction between language and communication has direct relevance to the functioning of deaf persons. As noted above, most deaf persons are adequate communicators using manual sign language, but are extremely retarded in their use of formal language skills (reading and writing). Many authorities do not consider manual sign language to be a true language, but rather an advanced communication system. A long-standing controversy among deaf educators revolves around the relative merits of oral versus manual techniques of communication and language learning; the issues are summarized in the following section.

Language and Communication Training Because deafness is synonymous with impaired language acquisition and reduced ability to communicate, language development and the training of communication skills have been the focus of educational programs for deaf children. Three basic approaches can be delineated: (1) the traditional oral method which stresses the skills of speech and speechreading; (2) the amplified hearing method which is premised on a developmental view of hearing, i.e., listening is a learned function; and (3) the total communication method which allows and encourages the use of fingerspelling and manual signs. Differences among these three approaches are, for the most part, a matter of degree, e.g., children trained under all three methods usually wear individual hearing aids and speech and speechreading skills are utilized by all three, but the degree of emphasis varies. Proponents of the three methods can cite evidence to support their favorite combination of techniques: DiCarlo (1964) writes convincingly of the traditional oral approach; Fry (1966) summarized arguments and presented data supporting the amplification approach; and Vernon and Koh (1970) reviewed and summarized a number of independent studies which favored the use of manual communication with deaf children. The only reasonable conclusion that can be reached at this time is that no method is appropriate for all deaf children. The importance of flexibility in the early language-communication training of deaf children cannot be overemphasized.

Most professional rehabilitation workers with the deaf share a definite bias for the manual approach to communication. This bias reflects the belief that a viable communication system which allows deaf children and youth to interact with their peers and to learn the basic skills which constitute maturity is preferable to a poorly mastered formal language system. More specifically, the bias reflects the experience of rehabilitation personnel in attempting to habilitate 20-year-old deaf adults who function socially as 10-year-olds. It is generally true that sign language restricts deaf persons to the deaf subculture, but this is viewed as the more desirable of the alternatives which are currently available. The issue is irrelevant anyway: most deaf persons associate with other deaf, join deaf social organizations, and intermarry.

Language and Intelligence Most traditional theories of mental development have been premised on the central assumption that language is the primary vehicle of intellectual development. The assumption of interdependence of linguistic and intellectual development has been fundamental in psychology, e.g., Carmichael (1957) concluded that "In a most important sense, the development of language in an individual is the growth of a human mind in that person" (p. 193). The implication is that mental development is retarded or distorted in the absence of language. As stated previously, investigations of the intellectual functioning of deaf subjects demonstrate that an individual's mental development is not dependent on the acquisition of language.

Investigations supporting the conclusion that intellectual development is independent of language development fall into three categories: (1) comparative studies employing experimental learning tasks (Furth, 1964; 1966; 1971); (2) comparative studies employing traditional (nonverbal) intelligence tests (Vernon, 1967; 1968); and (3) correlational studies using intelligence tests and language-communication assessments (Bolton, 1971*a*; 1971*b*).

The design of *comparative* studies is simple: matched samples of deaf and hearing subjects are compared on a variety of cognitive and perceptual tasks. Most comparative studies have concluded that there is no significant difference between deaf and hearing samples on learning tasks which do not require verbal mediation and, therefore, that language is not a necessary basis for abstract thinking and problem solving. Two points should be stressed: (1) many studies have found differences favoring hearing subjects, but these small differences reflect the cultural disadvantages and lack of "testwiseness" that penalize any minority group on psychological tests, and (2) strictly speaking, the conclusion is debatable because almost all deaf persons possess some minimal language skills (Blank, 1965; Bornstein and Roy, 1973).

The design of *correlational* studies of deaf subjects also is simple: a fairly large sample is assessed on several measures of nonverbal intellectual functioning, language abilities, and communication skills. The intercorrelation matrix of variables is factor analyzed to obtain the major dimensions of the intelligence-language domain. The results of correlational studies support and strengthen the conclusion reached in comparative studies: measures of language abilities define factors separate from the nonverbal intelligence factors.

Communication Skills The language-communication abilities of deaf persons are three in number (Bolton, 1973): (1) manual skills (manual signs and fingerspelling), (2) oral-verbal skills (speech and speechreading; reading and writing), and (3) residual hearing. Strictly speaking, residual hearing is not a language-communication modality. Furthermore, it is highly correlated with the development of oral communication skills, although it is only slightly related to measures of intelligence. A more important conclusion based on the results of several studies is that oral communication skills develop independent of manual communication skills and, therefore, that the early acquisition of manual skills does not impede the development of oral skills and may benefit linguistic development (see Bolton (1971a) and Vernon and Koh (1970) for a review of the research evidence).

Personality Development and Social Adjustment

It is generally recognized by child development specialists that a conception of selfhood becomes differentiated during the second or third year of life. The child's self-concept forms in the context of the socialization processes, which are inextricably correlated with language training and development. A question of importance to psychologists and educators concerns the extent to which personality development and social adjustment of the young child may be distorted by retarded language development. In the following sections several topics related to this question are addressed and, where appropriate, conclusions are drawn.

Personality Assessment   In contrast to the relatively straightforward evaluation of intelligence, achievement, and special abilities, the assessment of personality development and social adjustment of profoundly deaf persons is a difficult task. Generally speaking, standard personality inventories are not applicable to deaf persons. In addition to requiring a reading level of approximately sixth grade, standard inventories contain items which are not appropriate for persons with hearing impairments. Many projective instruments (e.g., Rorschach, TAT, etc.) are useful only with highly verbal deaf adults. Even with this small minority, the typical protocol is characterized by a paucity of responses with minimal elaboration. Most deaf adults lack the verbal facility to express their responses to unstructured stimuli. Finally, the traditional clinical interview relies to a great extent on verbal interchange between examiner and subject. When conducted by a psychologist fluent in manual sign language and experienced in work with deaf persons, the interview may provide useful information regarding personality functioning.

It is clear from the comments above that valid procedures for personality assessment of deaf children and adults are lacking. Therefore, all research studies are suspect and great caution must be exercised in interpreting results.

Personality Research   Six reviews of the research literature on personality and social adjustment of deaf and hard of hearing persons have been conducted during the last 20 years. Berlinsky (1952) reviewed 15 studies and concluded (pp. 49–50) that deaf persons appear to reach about the same overall level of adjustment as the hearing population. He then proceeded to enumerate "some slight but consistent differences." Deaf persons have more trouble adjusting to their environment, they are more introverted, less dominant, slightly more neurotic, slightly more ego-centric, evidence somewhat more feelings of depression and suspicion, and are less mature in judgment and social competence. Barker et al. (1953) presented a more critical review of essentially the same studies. They refused to draw any conclusions about personality or adjustment of deaf adults because of the inadequacy of the studies (p. 33). They concluded that deaf children in residential schools are more poorly adjusted, more unstable emotionally, and more neurotic than children with normal hearing (p. 33). DiCarlo and Dolphin (1952) reviewed more than a dozen studies of the personality and social adjustment of deaf children and adults and concluded that the results were inconclusive. They were especially critical of research design and measurement procedures employed in the studies. Meyerson (1963) considered the available studies of personality and social adjustment of deaf children and concluded that ". . . deafness is not directly related to personality in the sense that it requires a particular kind of adjustment" (p. 143). Levine (1963) reviewed a wide variety of studies and concluded that "the personality patterns and traits of the deaf . . . suggest weakness and deficiencies for dealing effectively and knowledgeably with the complex problems of life today" (p. 508). The final review by Schuldt and Schuldt (1972) considered 20 empirical personality studies of deaf children published since 1950. They concluded that deaf children manifest more abnormal personality characteristics and less adequate adjustment when compared to hearing children.

The reviewers are clearly not in agreement in the conclusions regarding the personality and adjustment of deaf persons. This may be caused by several factors, not the least of which is the diversity of methods and inconsistent results of the various studies. It is important to point out that all reviewers advised caution in interpreting their conclusions as indicating maladjustment or psychopathology. The question of practical concern remains: What reasonable conclusion can be drawn from the currently available studies of the personality and social adjustment of deaf children and adults? If it is assumed that ". . . what is normal or realistic for a hearing person may not be realistic for an individual who has impaired hearing" (Myklebust, 1964, p. 158), then the only defensible conclusion is similar to Levine's (1963) noted previously. Many deaf adults are deficient in the common knowledge and basic social skills that the average hearing person takes for granted. Most deaf persons grow up in a restricted environment and, consequently, they exhibit retarded behavior patterns. Generally speaking, these characteristics and conditions are responsive to educational-rehabilitative treatments as contrasted to psychological or psychiatric intervention.

Organismic Shift Hypothesis Many psychologists have hypothesized that any sensory deprivation produces an alteration of the pattern of sensory integration and a subsequent modification of behavior. Myklebust has been the foremost proponent of this notion in the study of the psychological effects of deafness. His "organismic shift hypothesis" is best stated by him:

> A sensory deprivation limits the world of experience. It deprives the organism of some of the material resources from which the mind develops. Because total experience is reduced, there is an imposition on the balance and equilibrium of all psychological processes. When one type of sensation is lacking, it alters the integration and function of all of the others. Experience is now constituted differently; the world of perception, conception, imagination, and thought has an altered foundation, a new configuration. (1964, p. 1)

Myklebust's explanation of the impact of organismic shift on the personality development of deaf children relies to a great extent on an intermediate cause, that of language deprivation. Again, in Myklebust's words:

> There is an assumption that deafness alters experience, that it causes an imposition on monitoring, and that it forces detachment and isolation. Furthermore, language is viewed as a significant factor in the development of personal-social contacts and interaction. Language is assumed to be the primary means whereby experience is internalized, crystallized, and structured. Hence, when language is limited there might be a reciprocal restriction in ability to integrate experience; the personality might be less structured, more immature, less subtle, and more sensorimotor in character. (1964, pp. 118–119)

There is no argument regarding the observation that many deaf youth and adults do exhibit retarded emotional development and personal functioning. What is disputed is the nature of the hypothesized cause; a much simpler explanation holds that deficits in experience are responsible for retarded personal-social functioning. The organismic shift hypothesis requires more confirming evidence before it can attain the status of an explanatory mechanism in the psychology of deafness.

Abilities, Interests, and Attitudes

Special Abilities Nonverbal abilities can be divided into two classes: (1) those which emerge primarily as a function of the maturational processes (e.g., spatial, clerical, and psychomotor abilities) and (2) those which require special training or exposure to certain activities and/or extended practice to stimulate optimal development (e.g., mechanical, artistic, and mathematical abilities). Deaf persons possess abilities of the first type in the same degree as hearing persons, but they often do not receive the requisite experiences to develop abilities of the second type. The psychologist who evaluates deaf clients should be careful to distinguish between tests which measure naturally developing abilities and those which reflect learning experiences.

Interests Interests develop in response to environmental stimulation and opportunities. Unlike abilities, the concept of interest requires an object of attention; interests do not exist apart from experience, which may be either vicarious or real. Because deaf persons are often not exposed to a wide range of educational and cultural experiences, their interests may be accurately described as underdeveloped. Thus, the measurement of interest patterns of deaf persons presents problems. Standard inventories such as the Strong and Kuder assume knowledge of activities which most deaf persons do not have. One of the several pictorial inventories which have been constructed, the Geist Picture Interest Inventory, was designed especially for use with deaf subjects. It has been demonstrated to be psychometrically deficient and clinically useless (Bolton, 1971c; 1972). Vocational guidance of deaf youth would be greatly improved by the development of a valid measure of interests.

Attitudes Two aspects of attitude toward deafness may be delineated: (1) the actual attitudes held by hearing persons, and (2) the attitudes that deaf persons believe that hearing persons hold (perceived attitudes). Both aspects of attitude toward deafness are potentially detrimental to deaf people: actual attitudes may result in real barriers to education, employment, etc., while perceived attitudes influence the deaf person's motivation and estimate of self-worth. The available evidence indicates that deaf persons devalue deafness more than hearing persons and that they believe that hearing people hold more negative attitudes toward deafness than they actually do. These conclusions have clear implications for educators of deaf children and youth, as well as rehabilitation counselors working with deaf adults. The interested reader is referred to Schroedel and Schiff (1972) for a review of the research evidence.

A CASE HISTORY

The case history which follows illustrates many of the principles of the psychology of deafness that have been reviewed in the previous sections. Paul was a client in the deaf project conducted by the St. Louis Jewish Employment and Vocational Service (JEVS). The case history is reprinted with permission from an article by Hurwitz and DiFrancesca (1968, pp. 262–264):

Paul is now a 21-year-old deaf boy who was admitted to the JEVS program at 19 years, 2 months of age. As a cerebral palsied child, he was unable to walk unassisted until age 5, when he first attended an orthopedic institute. Deafness occurred prelingually as a result of *meningitis,* which necessitated prolonged hospitalization. He retained a 75-db loss in his better ear and obtains some correction through an aid. His background is rural midwest, where his parents have always lived in modest but comfortable circumstances in a small community. He is the third child in a family of six children. His parents give the impression of a normally adjusted couple, devoted to home and family life. The father is a plant supervisor and the mother is a housewife.

At 6½, Paul's mobility was adequate for him to begin attendance at the state school for the deaf, where he continued his education until age 19, when he was discharged as having obtained maximum benefits. He did not qualify for an academic or vocational certificate. Academically he progressed only to a third-fourth grade level. He seemed to invest little in his school vocational training courses and failed to achieve even minimal proficiency in the several skills to which he was exposed.

On admission he was a tall boy, somewhat awkward in gait, and with facial and bodily residuals of his palsied condition. He was physically healthy and strong. Expression was through some intelligible speech and use of manual communication; reception was through a combination of residual hearing and speechreading or manual communication. His writing was extremely poor and he avoided this communication method wherever possible.

From observation and formal testing procedures, we learned these things about Paul: Moderate physical handicap was evident. His gross coordination was adequate for simple tasks but performance on tasks calling for fine muscle coordination was inferior. Some balance problem was evident. Communication was evaluated as well compensated in light of his auditory handicap and low language level. He displayed considerable initiative for freely communicating with both deaf and hearing persons. Cognitive organization was adequate; he could deal with task sequences and organize ideas into appropriate gestalts. Intelligence was in the normal range. No evidence of organic brain damage emerged from testing or behavior.

In personality, the boy was highly outgoing in an infantile manner, clinging verbally to others. His primary motivation seemed directed toward seeking and obtaining attention from others, primarily adults with whom he played the role of a good little boy. He was quite seductive in his appeal to adults, especially women. He displayed much fear of aggression toward others and was overly responsive to even mild criticism or mild rejection. While superficially sociable with peers he was obviously below his peer level in his interests (e.g., toward girls) and was unable to secure friendships. His primary emotional motivation was to secure adult attention and approval. A favorite means of gaining attention was by acting the clown. He would passively accept assigned tasks, but performance was extremely careless and perfunctory; task mastery and achievement had almost no intrinsic value for him.

Diagnosis Severe personality underdevelopment based on early physical trauma and disability and perpetuated by later oversheltering at both home and school, manifested by: infantile dependency on adults, repression of all affect that might disrupt dependency ties, competitive attitude toward peers, social development fixated at a very early age, and low level of independent task mastery. Social and emotional functioning was, in many respects, judged at a 3- or 4-year-old level. Positive attributes of intelligence, cognitive organization, capacity for interpersonal relationships, healthy affect, and aggressiveness all seemed favorable prognosticators for behavioral change.

Treatment Paul was treated in the JEVS intramural program for approximately 4 months and continued to receive ongoing assistance in the community for almost a year following employment. Since then he has obtained periodic help in problem solving when he has taken initiative to seek help. Intramural treatment consisted of a combination of traditional casework therapy techniques (ventilation, clarification, interpretation, and advice) and behavioral modification techniques that relied heavily on positive reinforcement of effective behaviors and extinction of inappropriate behaviors. It was found early that Paul, by contrast to many other clients, did have capacity for verbalization of feelings. A primary aim of the casework relationship was to seek the release and redirection of severely repressed hostile-aggressive feelings so as to free energies, now devoted to manipulation of adults, toward achievement of independent objectives. Not surprising for a boy who had once been so crippled he could not walk independently, he had enormous fear of bodily injury and he feared that his expressions of hostility would evoke destructive retaliation from others.

Simultaneous to counseling within a casework relationship, behavioral conditioning proceeded within the structure of his daily workshop regime and special efforts aimed at modifying bits of inappropriate behavior. For example, his enormous need for status and recognition was dealt with by offering him a job that would be uniquely his own and from which he could observe concrete, positive results, provided he performed his tasks punctually and accurately. This was the position of maintenance man, on whom many staff depended. Circulation around the agency also afforded great opportunity for attention-getting and dawdling. Clowning and prolonged inappropriate efforts to socialize with adults was handled by ignoring him; all staff were instructed to give him attention only during non-working periods.

Extinction of clowning and continuous talking slowly progressed and they remained in abeyance unless staff were manipulated into reinforcement of this behavior. Progress was sufficient to undertake job placement in a manufacturing plant, where he has since had a variety of jobs including stock work, messenger service, and even orientation of new personnel. Recurrent problems have been dealt with by directing industrial supervisors to apply those techniques that we earlier learned were effective and by supervising the implementation of these techniques. Despite dramatic improvements in self-sufficient behavior, he remained fixated in the belief that he could ultimately abandon responsibility for his own care and return home to a dependent status.

When he had, after 6 months of employment, demonstrated adequate work performance, the agency arranged for a family conference, in which his parents were encouraged to tell him explicitly that he would not be allowed to return home to live and that from then on he had to consider himself a self-supporting adult.

This conference marked the beginning of a conscious, though very reluctant, commitment to independence. Now, after 1½ years of independent functioning in the community, he is a proved employee. He continues to operate in many respects on a very childlike level: he is highly self-indulgent and saves no money from his very adequate wages; he attempts to elevate his self-esteem by outrageous lying; he is not capable of sustained friendships with peers and still relies heavily on older adult association. However, he is now committed to self-sufficiency and has proved capable of learning from many of his experiences.

FUTURE OF DEAF REHABILITATION

The purpose of this final section is to outline important services and discuss some issues relevant to the prevention of the potentially handicapping effects of profound deafness.

The origins of the problem, and thus, the key to the solution, are found in the parents' reaction to the diagnosis of deafness. After the diagnosis is made and confirmed (a process that usually occurs between 6 and 18 months after the child's birth), a sequence of (normal) emotional responses is manifested by the parents (see Mindel and Vernon (1971) for a thorough description). Professional intervention at this time is critical. Five topics related to the training and education of deaf children are discussed below.

Early Identification

Effective treatment and education of the deaf child require that the hearing loss be ascertained as early as possible. Normally, the mother will begin to suspect that something is wrong when the child is between 3 and 6 months old. The delay between initial suspicion and definitive diagnosis varies, but most congenitally deaf children are diagnosed by age 2 years. The use of infant screening procedures and the compilation of a high risk register can greatly improve the probability of early detection. All pediatricians should be trained to be attentive to indications of hearing defects in infants and be knowledgeable regarding referral sources.

Parental Counseling

The birth of a defective child precipitates a strong emotional reaction in parents. Shontz (1965) outlined a theory of reaction to crisis which includes five stages: shock, realization, defensive retreat, acknowledgment, and adaptation. The third stage, defensive retreat, which involves denial and the avoidance of reality, is critical for parents of deaf children. Because deafness is invisible and the diagnosis is made by inference, denial is relatively easy. Parental counseling requires psychological support during the early phases of emotional reaction following the diagnosis and accurate information during the phases of acknowledgment and reorganization. After the parents have worked through their feelings of disappointment and guilt and are ready to constructively prepare to deal with the task of raising a deaf child, they should be referred to educational specialists.

Communication Training

The reader now knows that deafness is synonymous with impaired language acquisition and reduced ability to communicate. Thus, language development and the training of communication skills have been the focus of educational programs for deaf children. The longstanding and bitter controversy between the oralists and manualists has made it virtually impossible for educators to provide an optimal language learning environment suited to the unique configuration of abilities and needs of each deaf child. The single most important quality of the early language-communication training of deaf children—flexibility—has been sadly lacking in most educational programs. There exists a critical need for research projects combining the best elements of the three language-communication teaching traditions.

Preschool Education

Approximately 90% of deaf children are born to hearing parents. Thus, only a small minority of deaf children are raised in an atmosphere in which deafness is a natural and accepted circumstance. Hearing parents require professional help to enable them to overcome their "disability" and provide a receptive and stimulating environment for their deaf children. (Deaf parents can also benefit from professional assistance.) Optimal preschool educational programs include: (1) formal training for parents so that they can learn to function as coeducators of their deaf children, and (2) preschool classrooms in which teachers especially prepared to educate deaf children direct a variety of activities designed to foster language and communication skills and enhance cognitive development. An innovative nursery school program designed and conducted at Michael Reese hospital in Chicago was described by Mindel (1969). A longitudinal follow-up study concluded that the intellectual and social development of 17 deaf children was comparable to or exceeded the establishment standards of normal development (Koh, 1972). The most recent statistics on preschool education of deaf children are encouraging: approximately 10,000 children under 6 years of age are enrolled in preschool programs and one-half of parents receive some kind of training related to their children's hearing loss (Office of Demographic Studies, 1972a).

Institutionalization

A large body of literature supports the widely held belief that institutionalization has detrimental effects on the developing child. One study which did not support this general conclusion compared matched samples of deaf residential pupils and day students attending residential schools (Quigley and Frisina, 1961). This investigation failed to support the contention that living in residential schools is detrimental to the development of communication skills, educational achievement, or the social adjustment of deaf children. For many deaf children, institutionalization is preferable to living at home where parents and siblings have never learned to communicate with them. A related issue is that of segregated versus integrated education. As noted previously, many studies of the personality and social adjustment of deaf children document their retarded development. This result is probably caused largely by growing up in a sheltered environment, isolated from the nondeaf world. Alternatives to attendance at a residential school (one-half of deaf children and adolescents attend them) are day schools, public school special classes, and regular classes. Integration into regular academic classes is feasible for deaf students with moderate hearing losses, excellent oral skills, and good psychological adjustment. O'Connor and Connor (1961) found that parent's interest and positive attitudes were related to their child's successful adjustment when they transferred to public school classes. Early identification, improved amplification, and widespread preschool education will enable a larger proportion of deaf children to enter regular public schools. But many profoundly deaf children will continue to require the special training that can only be provided in residential schools and day schools in metropolitan areas. Integration is still desirable in nonacademic subjects, vocational training, athletics, recreational activities, etc.

As more deaf children receive the benefits of preschool training and educational technology advances, a decreasing proportion of young deaf adults will become rehabilitation clients. But those who do will be the most severely handicapped and, thus, will require more intensive, long-term services. The overall net effect will be a continued shortage of appropriate services and professional rehabilitation workers for many years to come.

REFERENCES

Barker, R. G., B. A. Wright, L. Meyerson, and M. R. Gonick. 1953. Adjustment to Physical Handicap and Illness: A Survey of Physique and Disability. Revised Ed. Social Science Research Council, New York.

Berlinsky, S. 1952. Measurement of intelligence and personality of the deaf: A review of the literature. J. Speech Hear. Disord. 17:39–54.

Blank, M. 1965. The use of the deaf in language studies: A reply to Furth. Psychol. Bull. 63:442–444.

Bolton, B. 1971a. A factor analytic study of communication skills and nonverbal abilities of deaf rehabilitation clients. Multivariate Behav. Res. 6:485–501.

Bolton, B. 1971b. Factor analytic studies of communication skills, intelligence, and other psychological abilities of young deaf persons. Presented at the Psychometric Society meeting, April 8, 1971, St. Louis.

Bolton, B. 1971c. A critical review of the Geist Picture Interest Inventory: Deaf form: Male. J. Rehabil. Deaf 5 (2):21–29.

Bolton, B. 1972. A note on the Geist Picture Interest Inventory: Deaf form: Male. Rehabil. Res. Pract. Rev. 3(3):43–44.

Bolton, B. 1973. An alternative solution for the factor analysis of communication skills and nonverbal abilities of deaf clients. Educ. Psychol. Measurement 33:459–463.

Bornstein, H., and H. Roy. 1973. Comment on linguistic deficiency and thinking: Research with deaf subjects 1964–1969. Psychol. Bull. 79:211–214.

Carmichael, L. 1957. Basic Psychology. Random House, New York.

DiCarlo, L. M. 1964. The Deaf. Prentice-Hall, Inc., Englewood Cliffs, N.J.

DiCarlo, L. M., and J. E. Dolphin. 1952. Social adjustment and personality development of deaf children: A review of the literature. Except. Child. 8:111–118. Reprinted in E. P. Trapp and P. Himelstein (eds.), Readings on the Exceptional Child. Appleton-Century-Crofts, Inc. New York, 1962.

Fry, D. B. 1966. The development of the phonological system in the normal and the deaf child. In F. Smith and G. A. Miller (eds.), The Genesis of Language: A Psycholinguistic Approach. MIT Press, Cambridge, Mass.

Furth, H. G. 1964. Research with the deaf: Implications for language and cognition. Psychol. Bull. 62: 145–164.

Furth, H. G. 1966. Thinking without Language. The Free Press, New York.

Furth, H. G. 1971. Linguistic deficiency and thinking: Research with deaf subjects 1964–1969. Psychol. Bull. 76: 58–76.

Hurwitz, S. N., and S. DiFrancesca. 1968. Behavioral modification of the emotionally retarded deaf. Rehabil. Lit. 29: 258–264.

Koh, T. 1972. Cognitive and social development of postrubella deaf children of preschool ages: A follow-up study. APA Convention Proceedings, pp. 705–706.

Lerman, A. M., and G. R. Guilfoyle. 1970. The Development of Prevocational Behavior in Deaf Adolescents. Teachers College Press, New York.

Levine, E. S. 1963. Studies in psychological evaluation of the deaf. Volta Rev. 65: 496–512.

Meyerson, L. 1963. A psychology of impaired hearing. In W. M. Cruickshank (ed.), Psychology of Exceptional Children and Youth. 2nd Ed. Prentice Hall, Inc., Englewood Cliffs, N.J.

Mindel, E. 1969. Description of a preschool nursery for deaf children. In R. R. Grinker (ed.), Psychiatric Diagnosis, Therapy and Research on the psychotic deaf. (Final Report, SRS Grant No. RD-2407-5). Michael Reese Hospital, Chicago.

Mindel, E., and M. Vernon. 1971. They Grow in Silence: The Deaf Child and His Family. National Association of the Deaf, Silver Springs, Md.

Myklebust, H. R. 1964. The Psychology of Deafness. Revised Ed. Grune & Stratton, Inc., New York.

O'Connor, C. D., and L. E. Connor. 1961. A study of the integration of deaf children in regular classrooms. Except. Child. 27:483–486.

Office of Demographic Studies. 1972a. Characteristics of hearing impaired students under the age of six years: United States: 1969–70. Gallaudet College, Washington, D. C.

Office of Demographic Studies. 1972b. Academic achievement test results of a national testing program for hearing impaired students: United States: Spring, 1971. Gallaudet College, Washington, D. C.

Quigley, S. P., and D. R. Frisina. 1961. Institutionalization and psychoeducational development of deaf children. Research Monograph No. 3, Council for Exceptional Children.

Schiff, W., and S. Thayer. 1974. An eye for an ear? Social perception, nonverbal communication, and deafness. Rehabil. Psychol. 21: 50–70.

Schroedel, J. G., and W. Schiff. 1972. Attitudes towards deafness among several deaf and hearing populations. Rehabil. Psychol. 19: 59–70.

Schuldt, W. J., and D. A. Schuldt. 1972. A review of recent personality research on deaf children. In E. P. Trapp and P. Himelstein (eds.), Readings on the Exceptional Child. Revised Ed. Appleton-Century-Crofts, Inc., New York.

Shontz, F. C. 1965. Reactions to crisis. Volta Rev. 67:364–370.

Vernon, M. 1967. Relationship of language to the thinking process. Arch. Gen. Psychiatry 16:325–333.

Vernon, M. 1968. Fifty years of research on the intelligence of deaf and hard-of-hearing children: A review of literature and discussion of implications. J. Rehabil. Deaf 1(4):1–12.

Vernon, M., and S. D. Koh. 1970. Effects of early manual communication on achievement of deaf children. Amer. Ann. Deaf. 115:527–536.

2 | Language and Communication

HARRY BORNSTEIN,
JAMES C. WOODWARD, JR., and NORMAN TULLY

Unless you were born of deaf parents, it is unlikely that you will be able to communicate adequately with all of your deaf clients. Consequently, we will outline a variety of strategies which you can use to try to communicate better. None of the strategies is optimum. All will leave you with a more or less limited communication capability. And the sooner you are aware of this, the more realistic you will be about the quality of the service you provide the deaf client.

Before we can discuss strategy, we must first offer you a general description of language and some more specific descriptions of English and Sign. (We prefer to use the name Sign for what is often called the American Sign Language. It is short, accurate, and parallels the name for English.) Without these descriptions, you cannot really comprehend and effectively use the strategies we will discuss. You should further understand that linguistic descriptions of Sign have been developed only in the last decade. While there is a great deal more to learn about Sign, we have already learned much which is in direct contradiction to lay opinions and to most of the descriptions usually furnished by workers with the deaf.

Although deaf people are rehabilitation clients because of their hearing impairment, a substantial number, probably the majority, of them also have problems with English for the simple reason that most people learn English from hearing themselves and others. When they are unable to do this because of impaired hearing, they often achieve only a limited competence in English. Most deaf people have compensated for these limitations

19

in the spoken language by somehow acquiring a competence in a manual language. This creates an unusual, perhaps unique, counseling situation. Both you and your client may be language limited—he, in the auditory mode and, perhaps, in the written mode, and you in a visual mode.

Finally, this chapter will provide you with information which may help you deal with what may be one of the principal problems in communicating with a deaf client—your own ego. How will you accept and deal with your limitations when trying to communicate with a certain kind of client? As we outline the possible strategies for communicating with hearing-impaired people, you will further need to assess your own second language aptitude, your own motivation, and the amount of time you can afford to spend in trying to learn a visual language. As you will see, it is a most difficult and challenging assignment.

WHAT IS LANGUAGE?

General Facts

Let us first look at the complex phenomena called language. Most Americans, because of their culture, have grown up believing that there are right ways to speak and wrong ways to speak. This is a very culture-centered value judgment that sometimes approaches elitism and racism. A standard language is no better or more pure than a vernacular language. For example, double negative constructions, which are often considered modern illogical English, actually go back to old English kings like Alfred. Other languages, like Russian, negate everything negatable in a sentence so that a literal translation of one negative Russian sentence would look like: "He no when no thing not saw" or "He never saw anything."

The above literal translation looks like broken English, but be assured that using English grammar with Russian words is every bit as broken Russian. Thus, we are brought to a fundamental fact about language: every language has its own grammar. The closer a language is to another historically (English is closer to German than to Chinese), the more we can expect the grammars to be similar. As long as language even partially serves the needs of the people who use it to communicate, it will continue. When it stops serving those needs, it will not be used. Thus, judgments about the comparative worth of any language must be relative.

Each language has its own complexities and intricacies. If a language appears simple in one place, it may be extremely complex in others. Not everyone uses the same language in the same way. Language use varies on the basis of such social factors as age, sex, social class, race, ethnic origin, and many others. It must be stressed that language variation on the basis of sex and race (as well as other variables) is social, not biological. Women in American society tend to use a wider color vocabulary than men. Women apparently do not perceive differences in color differently from men, but they have more names for the differences than do men. That is, men may see the differences between two greens, but not label one lime and the other olive.

Variation, however, occurs not only in vocabulary but also in grammar and the sound system of a language. This type of variation is often stigmatized. Some Black American users of English are criticized for their lack of grammar when actually they are operating under some completely different rules from some White speakers. Some Southern speakers are castigated for sloppy pronunciation in not distinguishing *pin* and *pen,* while the critics sometimes do not distinguish between *caught* and *cot.*

It is extremely important for counselors to avoid negative attitudes toward language. For, no matter how openminded people are about other social groups, attitudes toward an individual's language can prejudice interaction.

This advice must be strictly regarded in relation to the deaf client, since deafness can be both a pathological and a sociological phenomenon. If a deaf client's English looks strange to a hearing person, such differences may or may not signify language incompetence per se. However, too often, hearing people, regardless of good intentions, overgeneralize about the abilities of some deaf people because of their English language limitations. The deaf person may be highly competent in another language that has almost always been ignored in education but not by some specialists and counselors in pastoral work—the American Sign Language or Sign.

Language Varieties of Deaf People

As previously noted, deaf clients may have a wide range of language competence. Apart from our knowledge of their English competence, there is, unfortunately, very little statistical information available on who uses the various sign language varieties. Linguists have yet to come to grips with this problem. However, it will be useful at this point to introduce some linguistic definitions of terms that will appear throughout the rest of the chapter. More detailed presentations of these terms occur later.

Fingerspelling Each of the individual letters of English words can be represented by separate hand configurations. Except for some special educational settings, fingerspelling is rarely used alone for communication, but is often combined with some variety of sign language.

Sign Language This includes any variety of signing that ranges along a continuum between Sign and Sign or Manual English. Each sign has a characteristic hand shape, position, movement, and orientation associated with it.

   Sign   This is the preferred language of the deaf community. As with many minority groups, deaf adults intermarry, socialize with each other in various ways, and are members of local, national, and international organizations. A common denominator for all of this is language and communication. It is not known how many deaf people there are who are not part of this community. Sign is not based on English, but is historically related to French Sign of the nineteenth century. Sign is more closely related to French Sign than British Sign, spoken English, or spoken French. Other names for Sign include American Sign language (ASL) or Ameslan.

   Pidgin Sign English (PSE)   This includes the intermediate sign language varieties on the continuum between Sign and English (Woodward, 1973). Pidgin English shares some of the characteristics of Sign and some of English, although some of the grammar of each language has been reduced. Pidgin Sign English is normally used in restricted formal situations and with hearing people by some members of the deaf community. Other terms for Pidgin Sign English include Signed English and Siglish.

   Sign or Manual English   These are systems contrived to represent English. Signs are used as if they were English words in English word order, as in Pidgin Sign English. Users of Sign English fingerspell or sign English word parts that are not present in Pidgin Sign English. Sign, or Manual English, represents "word parts" by spelling or newly developed signs. These systems are designed to represent English at home and in the classroom, e.g., Seeing Essential English (SEE 1), Signing Exact English (SEE 2), Linguistics of Visual English (LVE), and Signed English (Gallaudet Preschool System). These artificial systems have only one logical purpose: to enable the child to learn English. Thus, while some adult members of the deaf community may occasionally use PSE with fingerspelled endings in conversation with hearing people, almost no adult members of the deaf community will use (and many cannot understand) any of the artificial systems to communicate with each other. There would be no purpose served by doing so. Consequently, we will not discuss such systems further in this paper.

   Although Sign plays an extremely important role in the deaf community, it would be naïve to assume that all deaf adolescents or older adults are competent in Sign. Not all deaf people identify with the deaf community and with its major language, Sign. A survey of entering Gallaudet College students in 1968–1969 (Bornstein and Kannapell, 1969) found that only about one-half considered themselves fluent in Sign. About 15% judged themselves to have little or no ability. The same survey showed that 13% of them had learned Sign from parents, 63% from friends, and 37% from school staff. (Percentages add to more than 100 because of overlapping categories.) Fewer than 25% learned Sign before they were 5 years old. In all, about 60% learned before the age of 10 years. While this is not by any means a representative group of deaf adolescents, it would be surprising if backgrounds like these did not result in wide variations and competence in Sign. Perhaps the most striking of the statistics just cited are those which indicate that the most frequent source of knowledge about Sign came from friends at school. This is the most important difference between this language learning situation and those of other minority groups in the United States. Sign is most often *not* the language of the home nor of the neighborhood. In fact, it is usually regarded as a barrier between adult and child. Also, cultural achievements of the adult deaf community are rarely known to the hearing parents of deaf children.

In order to understand further the meaning of the extraordinary nature of the language environment of deaf children, we must briefly describe their home and educational situations.

About 90% of the deaf children in programs for the hearing impaired are born to hearing parents. Four percent of these children have two deaf parents and the remainder have one parent who has a hearing problem (Rawlings, 1973), The vast majority of hearing-impaired children, therefore, are viewed initially as medical problems by hearing parents and professionals. Quite naturally, these people are determined to overcome the child's impairment as much as possible. Simply defined, overcoming a hearing impairment has meant that the child develops competence in English and speech, makes optimum use of whatever residual hearing he has, and learns to speechread. Until this last decade, speech and competence in English were virtually regarded as synonymous. Competence in English, when achieved, was obtained through the medium of speech. The techniques used to achieve these desired results are highly structured, very arduous, and very different from those used with hearing children. These techniques, plus the necessary dependence on vision, sharply limit the amount of language to which the child is exposed. This reduction in language exposure probably accounts for some of the language problems of hearing-impaired children.

It has long been apparent that the great majority of hearing-impaired children achieve only a very limited degree of competence in English (Gentile and DiFrancesca, 1969). Recently the proposition that speech and language are synonymous has become increasingly suspect. First, the very existence of a manual language such as Sign suggests that speech and language can exist independently. Second, it also has long been obvious that deaf children depend in large part upon gestures and/or signs to communicate with other deaf children and with hearing adults *regardless* of the official communication practices of the school (Tervoort and Verbeck, 1967; Moores, McIntyre, and Weiss, 1972). Very simply, signs and gestures are a means of communication that will not disappear just to suit the wishes of educators and parents. Third, comparisons of academic performance of deaf children of deaf parents against those with hearing parents have favored the former without revealing any differences in speech. Since these children were exposed to a manual language early in life, many, if not most, educators of the deaf have considered anew the use of manual communication along with speech. An attractive name, total communication, appeared at just the right time to help further the use of manual communication. Unfortunately, total communication, as presently defined, merely allows for all types of manual signal without clearly specifying what kind of signal would be used for what purposes, with what kind of learner, and at what ages. It is quite clear that a long period of experimentation will be required before all of these questions will be answered satisfactorily.

The point of the foregoing paragraphs is to alert you to the fact that this is a time of rapid and significant change in the education of deaf children. The following descriptions may or may not be typical of those encountered years hence.

Deaf clients may be competent in Sign, English, both Sign and English, or neither Sign nor English. The sociological background, educational history, and the nature of hearing impairment of the client will have a great influence on which of these groups he falls into. Late onset of deafness, less severe hearing loss, sign language acquisition after the age of 6 years, and possibly other variables tend to indicate a person will have more English-like sign language competence and also more standard spoken and written English.

In general, early onset of deafness, profound hearing loss, deaf parents, or sign language acquisition before the age of 6 years, and perhaps other variables tend to mean that a person will have sign competence.

The language situation in the deaf community is a diglossic continuum between Sign and standard English. Diglossic situations are fairly common in hearing communities and occur in the spoken language situation in Arabic countries, Greece, Switzerland, and Haiti, to mention a few well-known examples. In diglossic situations, one language variety, generally a standard literary variety H, is in a special relationship with another language variety, generally a vernacular variety called L. H is used in more formal situations with more formal topics and with outsiders. L is used in less formal situations with insiders. H is often felt to be superior to L even by some native users, and some users will claim that L does not even exist. Acquisition of L is generally in the initial locus of enculturation; acquisition of H is in the formal educational system. H is studied in the schools; L is not. There are also large-scale grammatical works on H, and L is rarely if at all studied formally. Diglossic situations are typically very stable and may continue for several centuries.

The L language in the deaf community is Sign. Sign is a language in and of itself. It has a grammatical structure different from English and has little fingerspelling. For example, English—"Have you been to California?"—which is auxiliary, subject, verb, locational prepositional phrase, is translated into Sign as:

TOUCH FINISH CALIFORNIA YOU QUESTION

which is verb, auxiliary, locational noun, subject, and question, with subject and question signed simultaneously.

Sign has a number of highly interesting grammatical constructions. Instead of concatenations of inflectional endings, like many oral languages, Sign inflections are often internal modifications of the sign. This modification is found in such constructions as negative incorporation and agent-beneficiary directionality. In negative incorporation, the negative of a class of verbs is made by a bound outward twisting movement of the hand. In agent-beneficiary directionality, the relation between actor and receiver in a class of verbs is represented by movement in three-dimensional space from actor to receiver.

Reduplication is another common grammatical process in Sign. Reduplication in Sign, like reduplication in oral languages, may represent plurality of nouns, continuous action in verbs, or emphasis. Some other interesting grammatical characteristics of Sign include the nonexistence of a copula, the use of three-dimensional space to represent temporal, spatial, and pronominal relationships, and the use of the face, especially the eyes, to indicate constructions such as question, relativization, and pronominalization.

No complete grammar of Sign has been written, just as no complete grammar of any other language has been written. Researchers have only begun to scratch the surface of Sign syntax. What they have found is a highly complex and regular syntax.

In the deaf community, the H variety is normally Pidgin Sign English. An example of this is:

I FINISH BE RUN RUN

for English—"I have been running." "I" is an English pronoun, "FINISH" is a Sign aspect marker, "BE" is an English word that is signed (since there is no verb "to be" in Sign, this is purely English construction) and English "-en" has been deleted, and "RUN" has the "-ing" deleted.

The grammatical ordering of Pidgin Sign English then basically follows English word order. However, there is a reduction of English inflections and derivations, as one would expect of a pidgin, e.g., articles are variable, there is deletion of third person singular *s* on verbs, and the verb "to be" is not inflected. Some Sign grammatical constructions also exist in Pidgin Sign English, but they too are reduced. For example, the Sign verb "FINISH" functions for English "have" (nonpossessive). There is also the use of some, but not all, Sign agent-beneficiary directionality, negative incorporation, and verb reduplication. Pidgin Sign English generally has more Sign verb reduplication than negative incorporation and more negative incorporation than agent-beneficiary directionality. This by no means exhausts the grammatical characteristics, however. These characteristics were only chosen as a sample of the intermediate nature of Pidgin Sign English between Sign and English.

Because Sign and English are in close contact, they influence each other and tend to merge from their extreme differences into a continuum. Thus, all the regional, social, ethnic, and age varieties of Sign can be seen at one end of this continuum and all the regional, social, ethnic, and age varieties of English at the other.

The bilingual diglossic continuum between Sign and English that has been described is a phenomenon in the deaf community. Not everyone in the community can move freely and/or far along this continuum. Most members of the deaf community primarily identify with varieties approaching Sign and view Sign as the chief criteria for inclusion of members. A number of people can move somewhat toward Pidgin Sign English for formal conversations with hearing people. However, competence in a variety of Pidgin Sign English does not imply competence in the spoken and written English that almost all hearing counselors use. "Hearing" English, if learned at all, appears to be a second language for the majority of the deaf community. That is, many members of the deaf community do not have fluent command of the English language.

EGO COMPENSATORY BEHAVIORS
WHICH MAY OCCUR IN COMMUNICATION SETTINGS

We will restrict our discussion of ego compensatory behavior to those that may relate to language and communication. Observations are largely clinical in character because few data are available.

For the great majority of the hearing impaired, language and communication from the very beginning of life have been charged with tension and/or anxiety. Our lack of knowledge about manual communication in general and Sign in particular has been a fertile breeding ground for a whole range of practices which can hardly promote mental health. For example, until recently, it was often stated that a child who learned to sign, a seemingly easier task for the hearing impaired, could not be expected to persist in the difficult task of learning to speak and to lipread. (A few studies have compared the speech performance of children with manual backgrounds against those with oral backgrounds and found little difference.) This is a startling reversal of the usual practice of working from an easy to difficult task or from success to success. Moreover, schools have persisted in trying to teach speech and speechreading skills to the exclusion of manual skills until many children were in their teens. Then and only then were they permitted to sign.

It is these practices which are now being re-examined and, hopefully, changed. Until they are, it is easy to imagine the emotional background that a deaf adolescent might bring to a rehabilitation counseling situation. He or she is at that stage of life when his language skills in English and Sign may be among the most significant determinants as to which culture he may choose and/or be forced to live in. And the attitudes and emotions that others have displayed toward these languages and language skills can rarely, if ever, be separated from those skills. Indeed, as the following example suggests, some parents may reap a bitter harvest if they follow some "professional" advice. For example, a college student recently declared to the first author that if hearing parents really cared for the feelings of their deaf children, they would learn and use Sign (not Pidgin Sign English or one of the artificial varieties of signed English). She also asserted that her mother regarded her as some kind of strange creature because she could not speak well and, furthermore, that she had deliberately not learned to speak well as a means of getting back at her mother for not learning Sign.

Similarly, since hearing impairment is not visible and since deaf clients can often communicate well manually, one mechanism encountered is denial. In effect, some deaf clients will furiously reject any suggestion that hearing loss is an impairment or that, indeed, the client is different in any way. For example, the first author once received a furious letter complaining that the English text of a classical child's poem had been slightly altered. The writer's hearing grandchildren had unwittingly taunted him that deaf children were too stupid to learn the real poem. He had neglected totally the fact that the entire book was cast in a picture form of signed English and was as different from a conventional text as night from day.

There is, in addition, a type of reaction formation. Since many deaf acquire greater competency in Sign than in English, some may regard Sign as the superior language. Users maintain its superior effectiveness in all situations, including the academic. Furthermore, they regard it as the more beautiful language and capable of expressing more warmth than a spoken language. On the other hand, still other deaf persons have a love-hate relationship with Sign that has become very disconcerting to hearing people.

A skilled signer can manifest aggression toward hearing persons by speeding up his fingerspelling and signing, refusing to speak, or both. This kind of aggression can be expressed with or without awareness. Communication with counselors gives deaf people a rare opportunity to strike back, especially since it is they who are most often in difficult and sometimes frightening communication situations. We do not wish to overemphasize the frequency with which this last happens. In fact, it has been our experience that the reverse behavior is very much more common. More specifically, most deaf adolescents and adults can be and are incredibly gracious in trying to communicate with you provided that you have shown some interest in them and in their communication situation.

Additionally, many prelingually deaf adolescents and adults have a curious personal speech history. It is not uncommon to encounter a deaf adult who was assured and praised by his teachers on the adequacy of his speech, but who learned abruptly in the "real world" that his speech was actually barely intelligible and that his voice could cause surprise and, sometimes, distaste. Interviews of Gallaudet students taken about a decade ago revealed that many of them thought hearing people regarded them as animal-like because of their speech characteristics. It is not surprising that many of them deliberately do not speak rather than undergo the possibility of being further exposed to this kind of experience.

As noted in our introduction, the client is not the only one who will display ego compensatory behaviors toward communication with deaf people. Hearing people display their share, as well. Historically, the most characteristic one is the denial of Sign as language and its dismissal as an effective means of communication. In addition, hearing persons quickly and almost effortlessly pick up the ability to fake understanding when trying to communicate orally and/or manually. Just as deaf persons become embarrassed about their inability to handle the English language and/or their inability to read lips without error, so do hearing people become embarrassed in regard to manual communication. There appears to be some unspoken limit to asking people to repeat the same utterance. It becomes easier to let the "communication situation" continue on its course, even if some of the information really has not been received and comprehended.

There is one ego compensatory behavior, however, that appears to be more prevalent with hearing than with deaf people. It pertains to those who have learned to communicate manually. It seems to be easier for hearing people to learn to be productive manually than to learn to read or receive manually. It may be that the hearing person relies heavily on English syntax while transmitting Pidgin Sign English. In any event, it is very much easier to dominate a conversation transmitting "information" than to suffer with the uncertainties of reception. This may be particularly inappropriate in a counseling situation.

PROBLEMS IN COMMUNICATION
AND STRATEGIES FOR SOLVING THEM

One of the primary prerequisites of good counseling is good communication. This statement implies much more than a mere exchange of words between two individuals. Counseling, to be effective and beneficial to the client, must involve a true sharing of thoughts, ideas, and feelings. Unfortunately, this type of counseling is rarely available to deaf people. Far too often, counseling, if it is available at all, takes the form of a monologue rather than a dialogue, with the counselor doing the majority of the talking. Some of the reasons for this have already been described. Here we will deal basically with the inability of the counselor to circumvent the communication barrier imposed by deafness. This barrier is formidable and overrides and influences all aspects of the deaf person's life. "It is pervasive, deep, and resistant" (Switzer and Williams, 1967, p. 250). It does yield, however, to the counselor who is willing to adapt his usual means of communication to the needs of the deaf client.

The purpose of the discussion which follows is to present specific strategies which the counselor may employ in meeting the communication needs of his deaf clients. We wish to emphasize that these strategies are merely guides. If the resources you have available to you are limited, you will have to be as flexible as you can with these strategies.

In determining which method of communication is best suited for a particular individual, several points must be kept in mind. First and foremost is the principle that the deaf client should have the right to suggest the method to be used, and, second, the method may vary with an individual depending on the particular situation. A good practice for counselors to follow is to ask the client at the first interview how he wishes the communication to be structured. The client should also be encouraged to let the counselor know when he wishes to change the mode of communication.

The communication methods that are commonly used in counseling with hearing-impaired persons are speech, speechreading (lipreading), listening, writing, reading, fingerspelling, and one of the varieties of Sign language. These are often supplemented with natural gestures, pantomime, and the drawing of pictures.

The majority of deaf people tend to use Pidgin Sign English with hearing counselors and Sign with those deaf counselors who can handle it. For counselors unfamiliar with these methods, it is sometimes possible to utilize an interpreter in counseling situations. A small segment of the deaf population prefers the oral-aural method. This method utilizes speech and speechreading for communication purposes. Most hard of hearing individuals also seem to prefer this method. All hearing-impaired persons use writing, pantomime, and gestures from time to time in combination with the other methods.

Oral-Aural Method

The oral-aural method utilizes speech to send messages and speechreading, supplemented where possible with residual hearing, to receive communication from others. For a majority of hard of hearing people, as well as a small segment of the deaf population, this is the preferred means of communication.

While the oral-aural method requires only minor modifications in the way the counselor ordinarily communicates, it does present some special problems. For example, skill in speech does not automatically bring skill in speechreading or vice versa. When this happens, the counselor may find himself in the position of being understood by the client, but not understanding the client's attempts at communication. Or the reverse may occur, where he understands what the client is saying, but is unable to make himself understood. In such instances it may be necessary to supplement the oral-aural method with written communication. The fact that many speech sounds are not visible on the lips, or else can be confused with other sounds, also increases the possibility of misunderstanding. For this reason some writers have referred to speechreading as "educated guess work." Because of this problem it is not uncommon for some deaf people to act as if they understand when, in fact, they do not. To minimize this problem, the counselor should always check from time to time (without seeming to be interrogating or insulting) to be sure that he is being understood. (It is also possible to secure an oral interpreter, i.e., a person whose speech is more easily read than the average person's speech.)

Levine (1960) offers the following suggestions for communicating with the oral-aural deaf person:

1. The interviewer and the deaf individual should be seated facing one another and not more than 4 feet apart.

2. Light should come from behind the subject and be directed onto the interviewer's face. In this way light glare into the eyes of the lipreader is avoided, and he is free to concentrate in comfort upon the speaker's face.

3. The interviewer's speech should be natural, simple, and clearly enunciated, using whatever modifications in speed and volume are necessary for clearest comprehension. This can be established through brief experimentation. As a rule, the interviewer will find that his natural manner of speaking will not require much, if any, alteration.

4. To be avoided: grimacing, mouthing, shouting, speaking without voice, and marked slowdown in the delivery of speech. All of these distort mouth movements.

5. Also to be avoided: talking and smoking or chewing at the same time; resting cheek on hand; bending head, turning face away, and moving about while talking. All of these conceal or impair mouth movements.

6. Guard against fatigue on the part of the lipreader. A tired lipreader is not a successful one. When fatigue sets in, either pause for a rest or suspend the interview for the time being unless the subject expressly wishes to continue, possibly in written or manual communication.

7. Watch the face of the lipreader for signs of difficulty in comprehension. Puzzled expressions should be attended to immediately. Either the subject has not grasped a particular thought the interviewer is trying to convey or the vocabulary used has not been lipread successfully.

8. When difficulties in comprehension arise, clarification is made by rephrasing the concept or rewording the language into simpler and/or more visible forms, *but never by continued repetition.* Sometimes key words, expressions, and proper names that are particularly difficult to see on the lips may have to be written out.

9. When the interviewer is not sure a particularly important line of thought has been clearly understood, it should be expressed in several different ways and then discussed with the subject, and clarified further if necessary. Interviewers of the deaf are cautioned that understanding the single words of the vocabulary used does not always guarantee that the whole idea has been grasped by the interviewee.

10. Pads and pencils should always be available, one set for the subject and a set for the interviewer, with spare pencils in easy reach.

Suggestions for Understanding the Speech of Deaf Adults

In successful oral communication with deaf individuals, one side of the coin represents the lipreader's ability to understand the interviewer, but the other involves the interviewer's ability to understand deaf speech. The tones and inflection of deaf voices and the manner and rhythm of enunciation differ from normal utterance. In addition, there are individual variations in patterns of deaf speech, just as there are in the speech of the hearing. Some patterns are readily understood; others present difficulty.

1. When difficulties are encountered, a helpful procedure is to permit the deaf subject to talk uninterruptedly for a while to give the interviewer's ear a chance to become attuned to the particular tones and rhythm of the subject's speech. If the interviewer experiences embarrassment listening to uncomprehended speech, or if the subject has little to say, it is often helpful to request him to read aloud on one pretext or another. Having a known verbal context to which to refer helps the listener synchronize the sounds he hears with the words they stand for. During this auditory adjustment period, the interviewer should not strain for precise comprehension, but should rather open his ears to the general speech pattern until it finally sets into recognized verbal forms.

2. If auditory comprehension is still not achieved, the interviewer himself will have to resort to lipreading and watch the subject's mouth movements as skillfully as his own are being watched, combining what he sees with what he hears for comprehension. Whether aware of it or not, most hearing persons use a certain amount of lipreading among themselves. Those who work with the deaf find their natural abilities along these lines of great assistance in understanding difficult deaf speech.

3. When a deaf subject's speech cannot be understood through hearing and lipreading, written and/or manual communication will have to be used, depending upon the wishes of the subject and the abilities of the interviewer.

4. Occasional difficulties in comprehension arise even in the course of otherwise successful oral interviews. The interview should not be permitted to bog down on that account. A casual request to write out key words or expressions, or to repeat them, is not taken amiss by deaf persons. Or the interviewer can ask the subject to "tell me more about that." If understanding is still not achieved, the interview should continue never-

theless on the chance that clarification will come about in the course of further discussion. It usually does (Levine, 1960).

Paper and Pencil

In view of the many potential problems involved in the oral-aural method, it would seem logical to assume that the answers would lie in the use of written communication. This, however, is not the case. While some deaf people read and write exceptionally well, the great majority of deaf school learners read at around fifth grade level or below. Furthermore, writing is a slow and tedious method of communication at best.

Despite these limitations, paper and pencil communication can be a valuable tool in the hands of a skilled counselor. Some strategies for using this method of communication are as follows:

1. The counselor should avoid, whenever possible, the use of idiomatic and colloquial language, analogies, and complex abstractions. Some deaf people tend to interpret phrases such as "my head is spinning" quite literally. This can lead to considerable confusion. Always try to use simple vocabulary and short sentences.
2. Avoid, whenever possible, or at least attempt to clarify, words with multiple meanings, such as too, run, etc. It is not uncommon for a deaf person to understand a sentence like, "I *ran* to the store," but misinterpret the sentence "Mr. Nixon *ran* for president."
3. Where the written communication is not clear, the counselor should always attempt to get at the thought behind the words rather than the words themselves. This requires skill and patience but can be accomplished.
4. Do not assume that merely nodding one's head indicates understanding. Some deaf people may prefer to bluff their way through rather than suffer the embarrassment of admitting they do not understand. By tactfully asking questions which require the client to give back specific content, the counselor can determine if he is comprehending.
5. As noted earlier, always be prepared with pads and pencils for both counselor and client.

Fingerspelling

Most of the strategies discussed under written communication also apply to fingerspelling since fingerspelling is nothing more than writing in the air. Under some circumstances, spelled words (or abbreviations) "function" like signs. There are, however, certain differences between writing and fingerspelling which should be recognized. First, whereas written communication is permanent, fingerspelling is only temporary. With fingerspelling it is not possible to go back and re-read what has been misunderstood. Second, in normal usage, one does not pause for punctuation or capitalization in fingerspelling. Words run together and this makes for difficulty in reading. Third, and perhaps most important, a client's ability to comprehend English does not improve merely because print has been "transferred" from the page to the fingers.

Some strategies for helping to improve communication when using fingerspelling are:

1. When spelling, the hand is held in front of the body at chest level. Keep the palm of your hand facing the person you are speaking to and avoid undue movement with the hand. Try to think of your hand as a book which you are holding up for the other person to read. Moving the book up, down, or sidewise makes reading almost impossible.
2. Letters should be formed distinctly. Sloppy letter formation is comparable to slurred speech.
3. Try to maintain an easy fluid motion when moving from letter to letter with the wrist remaining in a relatively stationary position. Avoid spelling in spurts. A common problem for beginning spellers is to want to spell much too fast at the expense of rhythm and fluency.
4. When reading fingerspelling, try to visualize whole words and phrases rather than individual letters. This is difficult, but absolutely necessary if one is to read at a reasonable speed.
5. Avoid pretending to understand when, in fact, you do not. Deaf people will be considerate and slow down their spelling when they know the other person is experiencing difficulty.
6. Always be sure that the room lighting is adequate and that the deaf person is not facing a window. Fingerspelling for long periods can be very tiring on the eyes and, when looking into a glare, it can become doubly tiring.

Sign

Even though most of the deaf community is more comfortable with Sign than with Pidgin Sign English, there are still several reasons for believing that Pidgin Sign English will be more useful in counseling situations. Pidgin Sign English is closer to English than Sign and, therefore, will be easier (even though it will still be difficult) for the hearing counselor to learn than Sign. In fact, few hearing people appear to know Sign well. Also, because of the diglossic situation, deaf people expect that hearing people will approach English, that is, use Pidgin Sign English, rather than Sign. Finally, any type of signing on the part of a hearing person who has very little contact with the deaf community should elicit good rapport with a client who signs.

If the client is only competent in Sign, this will present the most communication difficulties between the hearing counselor and the deaf client, since it is very different from English. While an interpreter can be used, it is more difficult to find good interpreters for Sign because interpreters are hearing. Even if the interpreter has deaf parents, he will not necessarily be a truly effective interpreter of Sign. As with Pidgin Sign English, Sign interpreters may sometimes present more problems than they solve.

Use of Interpreter

Several problems arise when utilizing an interpreter in counseling situations. First, counseling, by its very nature, is an abstract process. When the deaf person is severely retarded linguistically in English and in Sign, as some are, the best of interpreters face a difficult, if not impossible, task in attempting to clarify messages between counselor and client.

A second problem has to do with the unique relationship characteristic of counseling. As noted by Vernon (1965), "The presence of an interpreter, regardless of his skill and sensitivity to the feelings of the deaf client and the therapist, is essentially an intrusion in this relationship" (p. 56).

Despite these and other potential problems, we feel that the interpreter can be a valuable tool working in cooperation with a skilled counselor. As a general rule, however, we would recommend that an interpreter be used only when no other means of communication is practical or when the client indicates that this is his preferred means of communication.

Several strategies which have proved helpful in utilizing interpreters are as follows:

1. Establish at the outset of the counseling session the roles of the counselor and the interpreter. This may appear obvious, but often is overlooked. Without this clarification, roles may become confused and the client may end up relating to the interpreter rather than the counselor. The interpreter should remain in the background as much as possible.
2. Never assume that the interpreter understands all that is involved in counseling and the client-counselor relationship. The problem of confidentiality is especially important since many deaf people are naturally concerned when a third party is involved.

3. Whenever possible, allow the client to select his own interpreter.

4. Avoid side conversation between the counselor and the interpreter. If problems develop which require discussion, these should be saved until a later time. Interpreters should never interject their personal opinions during a counseling session.

5. At the end of each counseling session check with both the client and the interpreter to see if any problems are developing. If these problems cannot be resolved, then consideration should be given to employing another interpreter, although this should be avoided if at all possible.

6. There may be times when two interpreters are needed, one deaf and one hearing. This might occur when the client could only communicate with a deaf interpreter. Again, the roles of all parties involved must be clarified.

7. Whenever possible, avoid the use of English idiomatic expressions. Although a qualified interpreter can usually change these expressions into language which is familiar to the client, the danger of misinterpretation is always present.

8. Encourage direct communication between the counselor and client whenever possible. In some instances the interpreter may be needed only to clear up some confusion.

9. Always have the interpreter seated close enough to the counselor so that the client can see both of them with ease.

10. Before the first counseling session the interpreter should meet with the deaf client in order to determine what language variety the deaf client prefers.

11. Never assume that all deaf people will want an interpreter. Some deaf people would prefer to do their own communicating regardless of the difficulties involved. Others, from oral backgrounds, may wish to have an oral interpreter. This latter group may have strong feelings against manual communication and feel insulted if Sign were employed.

12. All communication should be directed to the client (e.g., use "you") even though it is the interpreter who may be speaking for the client.

13. The counselor should continually observe the facial expression and behavior of the client even while his remarks are being interpreted.

14. The counselor and interpreter should avoid facial expression which might convey false or undesirable impressions to the client.

If you wish to obtain the services of a manual interpreter or learn Sign, you can contact the Registry of Interpreters for the Deaf, Inc., P. O. Box 1339, Washington, D. C. 20013. The telephone number is (202) 447-0511. The RID has a national evaluation program for its members and awards certificates for competence in interpreting skills. For a nominal fee, you can secure a directory which lists members by state. The Communication Skills Program of the National Association of the Deaf, 814 Thayer Avenue, Silver Spring, Md. 20910, will also help set up courses in Sign.

RESOURCES FOR LEARNING MANUAL COMMUNICATION

If you decide to try to acquire some skill in manual communication, there are a variety of options open to you. However, you should know that you will probably have to rely on your own taste in your final selection of materials. There are almost no data which you can use to help you choose one set of materials over another.

The task of learning signs and/or fingerspelling is usually broken down into two phases: (1) recognizing and being able to execute isolated signs and (2) receiving and transmitting connected discourse for one or another of the Pidgin Sign English varieties described in this chapter. The vast majority of materials available place great stress on vocabulary acquisition and provide almost no information on syntax. Indeed, most books are simply Sign lists. The reader is given English word order to follow as if that is the way signs are ordered. There may be an occasional reference to multiple meanings of some of the signs and some features of English which are not present in Sign, e.g., the absence of articles. But that is all that the reader will learn about this unusual language.

Until just the last few years, all of the materials on Sign have been prepared knowingly or unknowingly for the hearing adult. That is probably the principal reason they are in Pidgin Sign English. It is difficult to find a deaf adult who deals with these materials with any purpose other than to teach hearing adults. (Ironically, those who advocate standardizing or specifying "acceptable" signs invariably wind up proposing a format, usually a book, only used by non-native signers. The process is analogous to preparing a book on English for Americans, selling the books to immigrants, and then expecting the book also to serve as the standard for native speaking Americans.) A major consideration in the preparation of materials is cost. When signs are presented, they usually are presented pictorially. This is expensive, whether by static picture, film, or videotape. It is this cost which is probably a major reason why such materials have had limited success. More specifically, it is exceedingly expensive to create enough practice material for a learner to reach an acceptable level of performance.

There are two general sources that you can use to locate most available materials. The first is the appendix of *A Basic Course in Manual Communication* (O'Rourke, 1973) published by the National Association of the Deaf

(NAD), and the second is a catalog of training films and other media for special education published by the Educational Media Distributing Center, Conference of Executives of American Schools for the Deaf, Inc. This latter organization makes materials available on a free loan basis to groups that are registered with the Media Services and Captioned Films Program. Registration may be accomplished by writing to the Center at 4034 Wisconsin Avenue, N.W., Washington, D.C. 20016, describing briefly the program for which the materials are desired. There are at least two sets of materials available from this source that will be described later.

The appendix of *A Basic Course in Manual Communication* attempts to include all materials made since 1966. Each item is described by at least several paragraphs. Sometimes evaluative comments are made, but not every item is so treated. The materials cited are those which are offered commercially. Many are included on the NAD publication list.

There exists also a very sizable amount of instructional material which has been prepared by schools, church and social work organizations, and universities. In truth, we do not know if there is any significant difference in quality between these materials and those listed in the two sources already cited. It would seem very desirable if a register were established that would provide a comprehensive description of these materials. Meanwhile, your own intuition and "expert opinion" are the principal guides to choosing materials in this area.

We will turn now to the specific techniques you might use. First, let us consider fingerspelling. You can learn to form and to recognize the 26 letters of the alphabet in about 1 hour. In a matter of several weeks at your convenience and without other materials you should be able to transmit letters at a rate which might be half that of an experienced speller. Very experienced spellers can comfortably and intelligibly spell at approximately 40% the rate of normal speech (Bornstein, 1965). Usually, it is very much more difficult to learn to read spelling than it is to transmit. Reading spelling is further complicated by the fact that words will usually be spelled to you in the midst of a stream of signs. If you stick to spelling alone, then a machine is surely the best way to learn it, and the Media Services can provide you with two fingerspelling series. Series I has nine lessons or cartridges, and Series II has a set of 11 cartridges. No information is available on the skill you can reach with these materials, but results obtained with hearing undergraduate students on an experimental course in reading the manual alphabet suggest that such skill is limited. In that study (Bornstein, 1965), subjects, after an average training time of 13 hours and 40 minutes, were able to read a modest number of discrete words spelled at moderate speeds. They were not able, however, to read an appreciable number of spelled sentences correctly. The study also failed to demonstrate that learner control over rate of presentation substantially affected learning. In addition, responding orally, in writing, or manually to the film also failed to show any practical differential effect on learning. In short, if you practice diligently, you will acquire a very limited capability to read fingerspelling.

As noted above, the considerable amount of instructional material on manual communication that has been prepared over the last decade, regardless of title, deals almost exclusively in Pidgin Sign English. Early in this period, the usual type of material consisted of a dictionary of signs which would serve as a course text or reference. In these books, signs are most often drawn, sometimes photographed, and/or described in words. The number of signs varies from about 500–1000. Invariably, one or two English "equivalents" are associated with a sign. Regional and ethnic variation in Sign is almost never noted. Exercise materials, where supplied, are almost always in English syntax.

Hoemann and Hoemann (1974) have demonstrated that "naïve" subjects can execute correctly 87% of a set of signs from merely looking at line drawings supplemented with word descriptions. They further note some ways the drawings and word descriptions could be improved which suggests that the percentage of accurate executions could be still higher. With a little experience, therefore, you should be able to execute almost any sign reasonably well from seeing it drawn and described on paper. In short, consulting a book is a reasonable *start* to acquiring skill in executing discrete, unconnected signs. This is somewhat equivalent to having a large French vocabulary without having any knowledge of how to put it all together.

The formats of the most recent works are much more varied, attractive, and ingenious. These consist of flashcards, playing cards, overlays, motion picture films, and videotapes. Some of these newer materials are designed to be self-instructional. Film courses are shown through use of 8-mm cartridge projectors. A few courses run as long as a few hours in segments of 5 minutes each. One videotape series offers as much as 13 hours of material in ½-hour segments. A few of these films show some expressions that are characteristic of Sign and begin to introduce the learner to sign order which is different from that of English. Without doubt, such self-instructional materials are more expensive than texts. They also serve to develop some degree of skill, but it is also clear that none takes the learner very much beyond a beginner's level in receptive skill, if that far. But even that is a considerable accomplishment.

Only one work treats signs as Sign (Fant, 1973). Using a basic vocabulary of 400–500 signs, the text and associated films attempt to convey meaning within Sign syntax. There is a second text that treats Sign expressions and structures within a general English syntax (Madsen, 1972). The language complexity of this Pidgin Sign English work is considerably higher than that of the previous work. All of the works so far described work with vocabularies of less than 1,000 signs.

If recent materials are any indication, it seems very likely that instructional material will continue to increase in sophistication and provide an even better means to learn manual communication. There are certain areas in which we believe considerable development is both possible and desirable.

1. Instructional materials directed at teaching Sign or a Pidgin Sign English close to Sign should go beyond the core 500–800 signs currently found in such works.
2. A shift in general approach in presenting Sign and English "equivalents" might be helpful for hearing people. As noted above, one, occasionally two, English "equivalents" are generally offered to define a pictured Sign. These Signs are usually grouped in semantically related units. In essence, the English words are keyed to the Sign. If this were reversed, if the pictured Signs were keyed to English words or phrases, hearing learners might derive an altogether different perception of Sign. For example, it can be shown that several signs in different situations are often used by deaf persons to translate in Sign or parallel in Pidgin Sign English a given English word.
3. The organizational principles followed in *A Dictionary of American Sign Language on Linguistic Principles* (Stokoe, Casterline, and Croneberg, 1965) might suggest simple and efficient ways by which individuals can look up English equivalents to Signs encountered in daily life.
4. Some of the logic and techniques used in the patterning exercises developed for second language teaching purposes should be transferable. It could be especially helpful in teachiing Sign grammar.
5. Sign is not simply a succession of individual Signs. It has a grammar which is based on very different principles from English, as we have already shown. Instructional materials can and should be developed to teach explicitly these aspects of Sign to hearing people.

In the final analysis, you are unlikely to acquire a reasonable degree of competence in Sign or Pidgin Sign English without extensive interaction with users of the language. This calls for a considerable investment of your time and an active and continued effort to meet with deaf people in a variety of settings. In all probability, you will have to expend as much effort as you would to learn any other second language. Competence is not easy to come by.

REFERENCES

Bornstein, H. 1965. Reading the Manual Alphabet. Gallaudet College Press, Washington, D. C.

Bornstein, H., and B. M. Kannapell. 1969. New Signs for Instructional Purposes. Final report OE 6-1924. Gallaudet College Press, Washington, D. C.

Fant, L. J. 1973. Ameslan—An Introduction to American Sign Language. National Association of the Deaf, Silver Spring, Md.

Gentile, A., and S. DiFrancesca. 1969. Academic Achievement Test Performance of Hearing Impaired Students in the United States: Spring 1969 (Series D, No. 1). Office of Demographic Studies, Gallaudet College, Washington, D. C.

Hoemann, H. W., and S. A. Hoemann. 1974. Pictorial and Verbal Representations of the American Sign Language Lexicon. American Psychological Association, New Orleans, La.

Levine, E. S. 1960. Psychology of Deafness. Columbia University Press, New York.

Madsen, W. J. 1972. Conversational Sign Language II. Gallaudet College Press, Washington, D. C.

Moores, D., C. McIntyre, and K. Weiss. 1972. Evaluation of programs for hearing impaired children. Report of 1971—72. Research report 39, University of Minnesota, Minneapolis, Minn.

O'Rourke, T. (ed.) 1973. A Basic Course in Manual Communication. National Association of the Deaf, Silver Spring, Md.

Rawlings, B. 1973. Characteristics of Hearing Impaired Students by Hearing Status, United States: 1970—71, Series D, Number 10. Office of Demographic Studies, Gallaudet College, Washington, D. C.

Stokoe, W. C., Jr., D. C. Casterline, and C. G. Croneberg. 1965. A Dictionary of American Sign Language on Linguistic Principles. Gallaudet College Press, Washington, D. C.

Switzer, M. E., and B. R. Williams. 1967. Life problems of deaf people. Arch. Environ. Health, 15:249—256.

Tervoort, B., and A. Verbeck. 1967. Analysis of Communicative Structure Patterns in Deaf Children. V.R.A. Project RD-467, 6465 (Z.W.O. Onderzoek, NR: 585—15). Groningen, The Netherlands.

Vernon, M. 1965. Interpreting in counseling and psychotherapeutic situations. In S. P. Quigley (ed.), Interpreting for Deaf People, pp. 94—104. U. S. Department of Health, Education, and Welfare, Washington, D. C.

Woodward, J. 1973. Some characteristics of pidgin sign English. In Sign Language Studies, Vol. 3, pp. 39—46. Moulton, The Hague.

3 | Intellectual Development

HARRY W. HOEMANN
and **DOUGLAS G. ULLMAN**

When rehabilitation counselors work with deaf clients, a frequently asked question is: of what value is the IQ score which is generally included in the report from a psychological evaluation? Although an index of intellectual functioning, such as an IQ score, is often helpful in rehabilitation planning and counseling with many clients, there is considerable question as to whether the IQ score obtained by deaf individuals adequately reflects their intellectual development or functioning. On most commonly used verbal tests of intelligence, it has been reported that the mean IQ of deaf persons is from 5—15 points below the mean IQ of the general population with normal hearing (Sattler, 1974). When nonverbal IQ tests are used, the picture is somewhat different, as about half of the studies find a similar relative deficit for the deaf, but the other half of the studies report either no differences or, in some cases, a relative superiority for the deaf (Meyerson, 1963; Sattler, 1974). When IQ differences are obtained, there has been extensive debate over whether these differences are the result of differences in intelligence or the result of a variety of other factors.

There appear to be two diverging viewpoints regarding intellectual development in deaf persons. On the one hand, the developmental lags

The preparation of this report was supported by National Institutes of Health Research Grant NS-09590-05 from the National Institute of Neurological Diseases and Stroke.

that have been observed on a variety of cognitive tasks combined with the deaf child's proverbial language deficit are often cited as a clear indication that a cognitive deficiency typically accompanies deafness. On the other hand, the extent to which large numbers of deaf adults manage their public commitments and their private lives with poise and confidence can be cited as evidence that intellectual functioning is not necessarily impaired seriously by deafness and that it is inaccurately measured in deaf persons by traditional methods.

We propose to clarify some of the issues which are implied by each of the above positions. We intend to relate information on intellectual development in deaf persons to unavoidable theoretical issues, including what intelligence is and how it is to be measured. Then we will discuss how these issues interact with deafness when intellectual development is assessed by traditional IQ tests and by a variety of experimental means. Finally, once the measurement of intelligence is reduced to an operation which is open to frank discussion, we hope to provide professional persons who work with deaf clients a rationale for using information derived from tests of intelligence, school achievement, and other sources that is not only theoretically defensible but also soundly practical.

WHAT IS INTELLIGENCE?

Human intelligence is often contemplated with a certain amount of awe, as if it were a mysterious, elusive "something" which everyone has, but which some people have more of than others. This mystique is often fostered by the secrecy surrounding IQ test scores and by the professionalism which characterizes test administration. Schools and clinics typically do not disclose IQ scores either to the client who was tested or to the general public. This policy is intended as a safeguard against the misinterpretation of IQ test scores or the inappropriate use of IQ test results. Moreover, if tests must be administered properly for their results to be reliable, it makes good sense to insist that only trained and experienced examiners be allowed to administer them.

Unfortunately, as with many well intentioned policies, concerns over the confidentiality of IQ scores and over the qualifications of examiners have sometimes had unfortunate side effects. The cloak of secrecy surrounding IQ connotes an artificial elitism, as if only certain persons had been initiated into the secret rites and the rest of society had to stand outside the inner sanctum. The professionalism which is aimed at protecting society from untrained and inexperienced test administrators has further emphasized the division between the "elite" and the public.

It needs to be emphasized that it is their conservatism that prompts specialists in testing to be somewhat guarded in their manner toward IQ tests and IQ scores. While they have every right to be proud of their achievements in constructing tests which measure individual differences, they do not wish to misrepresent the product they have made possible. In good hands, a carefully selected test, properly administered, can provide very useful information for those who have been trained to use it appropriately. Anything short of that set of circumstances is likely to lead to abuse. It is to protect both the public and the individual client from such abuse that test construction and test administration are surrounded by certain professional safeguards.

Definitions of intelligence generally betray theoretical biases. Individuals who are committed to the position that there are strong genetic determinants of intelligence typically describe it as the ability to learn or a capacity to adapt. They generally assume that such ability or capacity is largely innate. In contrast, individuals who prefer to think of intelligence as a product of experience tend to describe it in terms of what a person has learned or the strategies for processing information which he has acquired. Although neither position forces a conclusion as to the extent to which intelligence is fixed, there seems to be a tendency for people who believe it to be innate to also believe that it is relatively unchangeable and for people who believe it to be acquired through experience to believe that it is highly modifiable. Alternatively, those with a more pragmatic viewpoint define intelligence as whatever it is that IQ tests test. While this position may have some practical advantages, it depends heavily on the established correlates of IQ tests for the general population and is, by its very nature, circular.

A relatively neutral definition of intelligence has also been ventured from time to time which calls attention to problem-solving ability or to the abstract thinking ability of individuals. There seem to be clear individual differences in the ability to solve problems and to think abstractly, with better performances coming from those who can be presumed to be more intelligent. This kind of definition has an initial advantage in that it leaves open the questions addressed previously, namely, whether this ability is innately given or whether it is acquired as a function of experience, and whether it remains relatively constant throughout one's life or whether it can be improved by training or instruction. However, as with the pragmatic definition, the relative advantages of this one are somewhat costly, since they are gained at the expense of suggestions as to what the determinants of intelligence might be or how they might interact with one another during the course of development.

Regardless of the theoretical bias, or lack of one, that characterizes definitions of intelligence, there are certain commonalities which cut across all of the positions and on which scholars are, for the most part, united.

1. It is assumed that there is an innate capacity in individuals which sets limits on what they can do. This innate capacity is considered to be a part of one's genetic endowment. Individuals are believed to differ from one another in terms of their innate capacity.

2. Whether an individual fully achieves the optimum intellectual levels associated with his genetically determined potential depends on a number of environmental factors. Any physical or psychological damage, whether prenatal, perinatal, or postnatal, may detract from the extent to which one's potential will be realized. For example, the effects of malnutrition on intellectual development have been well documented, and it is widely believed that intelligence will not develop optimally in an unstimulating environment.

3. There is considerable consistency in individual human behavior across time. Thus, a person who was precocious at age 6 years will probably be higher than average in intelligence at 16, and a person who was retarded at age 6 will probably be lower than average in intelligence at 16. The "probably" is an important qualifier, however, since inferences about precocity and retardation have sometimes been mistaken. Moreover, abilities become more complex with development; consequently, one cannot always predict from ability at a very young age what will be the case at a more mature level of development.

4. There is considerable generality in individual human behavior across tasks. Thus, a person who performed intelligently in one situation will probably perform intelligently in another and vice versa. This generality of intellectual functioning is reflected in Spearman's position that a single factor accounts for most of the variance in a battery of tests designed to assess intelligence. It also supports definitions of intelligence such as Wechsler's "global capacity." There is some disagreement, however, over the issue. Other specialists, like Thurstone, have theorized that intelligence is comprised of a number of relatively independent abilities which develop concurrently.

Again, the "probably" in the preceding paragraph is an important qualifier. Not all failures are indicative of low intelligence. Poor performance or failures in a specific situation may result from a variety of psychological or physiological factors which are unrelated to intelligence. For example, certain kinds of neurological dysfunction may affect specific behaviors, such as reading, without necessarily implying inferior ability at reasoning or problem solving. Early profound deafness typically precludes normal acquisition of linguistic competence in a spoken language, and deaf persons typically earn low scores on tasks administered through verbal instructions or which require a verbal response. At the same time, deafness does not preclude a high level of performance on nonverbal tasks.

But if failure in certain tasks is sometimes misleading, so is success. There are instances in which phenomenal abilities of a certain kind, such as mathematical reasoning or memory for certain kinds of information, may occur in persons whose intelligence is average or even retarded in other respects. In fact, autistic children, who lack normal adaptive behaviors relative to other persons, may manifest highly intelligent behaviors in specific classes of tasks.

5. It is widely conceded that intelligence tests do not give us a privileged glimpse at raw, innate ability. They are performance measures. As such, they depend on the interaction of genetic factors and the individual's environment and experience. Since they were developed within the context of an educational setting, the best predictive power of the IQ tests is for performance in school. As indicated earlier, there is considerable question as to whether IQ tests adequately reflect intellectual development in the minority elements of a society, such as the deaf. However, independent of this question, there is little disagreement that such tests do, in general, predict relative success in school settings designed for the majority of the population. While this information may be of some value in and of itself, there is virtually no information available on whether IQ tests will predict relative success by minorities in other types of settings, such as other types of school settings, job performance, marriage and family life, social adjustment with peers, etc. It is not surprising, therefore, that some people refer to IQ tests as types of scholastic aptitude tests.

DEVELOPMENT OF INTELLIGENCE TESTS

The carefully developed intelligence tests that are likely to be used by trained examiners today are the culmination of over 70 years of experience in test construction. Modern intelligence tests have a number of European roots, including work done in the experimental psychology laboratory founded by Willhelm Wundt in Leipzig, Germany, and the programmatic research project on heredity carried out under the direction of Sir Francis Galton in England. However, the principal originator of intelligence tests as we know them was a Frenchman, Alfred Binet, who was charged with the responsibility for identifying mentally retarded children for the French Minister of Education. Binet tried a variety of approaches, some of which were simple measures of tactile, auditory, or visual acuity and of reaction time to the onset of a stimulus. Galton and Wundt were optimistic that this strategy would eventually lead to a measure of intelligence. It made good sense if you subscribed to the philosophy of John Locke, who believed that knowledge entered the mind through sensory experience. The better one's sensory abilities, the more the mind could take in and, therefore, use to act intelligently. Unfortunately, things turned out to be not that simple. Binet began to suspect this, and he and his colleague, Simon, included complex tasks involving memory, problem solving, and abstract thinking in their test battery. By 1905, Binet and Simon were able to assemble a series of 30 tests arranged in order of difficulty which could differentiate more and less intelligent children by the number of tests that the children passed. Binet died an untimely death in 1911, but before he died he had played a major role in developing a test of intelligence which had predictive validity in the Paris schools.

The 1908 and 1911 versions of the Binet-Simon test made use of the concept of a mental age. If a 10-year-old child passed all of the tests that were typically passed by a 10-year-old child, then he was said to have a mental age of 10. If he passed all of the tests that were typically passed by a 12-year-old child, he was said to have a mental age of 12. By the same token, if he only passed all of the tests that were typically passed by an 8-year-old child, and none higher, he was said to have a mental age of 8. The Binet-Simon tests were translated into English by Terman at Stanford University. They have become known as the Stanford-Binet Intelligence Test. The first version, published in 1916, made use of a point scale similar to that used by Binet and Simon. The 1916 version first made use of the concept of an intelligence quotient. The mental age was divided by the chronological age and multiplied by 100 to yield scores which were reported to measure the rate of mental growth. The previously mentioned 10-year-old child with a mental age of 12 would have an IQ of 120, while the 10-year-old child with a mental age of 8 would have an IQ of 80. An IQ of 100 is considered to be normal, since it reflects a mental age that is developing at the same rate as the chronological age. There was a major revision of the Stanford-Binet Test in 1937. Knows as the Merrill-Terman revision, it was standardized on a relatively large number of children compared to the earlier versions and to other tests on the market. In addition, considerable effort went into developing items which correlated with the total test. Alternate forms, L and M, were prepared so that one administration would not spoil a subject for retesting shortly afterward.

This was a favorite instrument among clinical psychologists for many years.

There was another major revision in 1960, but the changes did not affect the type of test items that were used. In the 1960 version there are no longer two forms; instead, the best items from both forms were combined into a single instrument. It still resembles the earlier versions in content, and the procedures for administering it are similar. The result is still reported as an IQ score, although it is no longer derived as a quotient, MA/CA. Instead, norms have been developed for each age, and deviations above and below the mean score typical of each age are transformed into IQ scores. Since deviation IQ's are derived statistically, it is possible to arrange that the same amount of variability is associated with the IQ score regardless of age level. In the case of the 1960 Stanford-Binet, the standard deviation is 16. Theoretically, IQ scores are normally distributed. This means that the normal curve can be used to derive proportions of the population that are likely to obtain scores as high as or higher than individually specified values. For example, a score of 132 is two standard deviations above the mean. Fewer than 2½% of the population would be likely to score as high as 132.

In 1972, the norms were updated and included a better sampling of minorities. The changes were relatively minor and did not change the way in which intelligence was conceptualized or measured.

The best known competitors of the Stanford-Binet are the Wechsler scales, developed by David Wechsler at Bellevue hospital in New York. Wechsler criticized existing tests for being inappropriate for adults and for overemphasizing verbal ability and speed. The Wechsler-Bellevue Intelligence Scale, published in 1939, was developed explicitly for adults. A revised version, known as the Wechsler Adult Intelligence Scale (WAIS), appeared in 1955. It consists of 11 subtests, six of which contribute to a verbal IQ score and five of which contribute to a performance IQ score. The six subtests on the verbal scales are so named because they all require the client to verbalize his answers. On the other hand, the five subtests on the performance scales do not require the client to produce verbal answers. There is also a full scale IQ, which reflects the client's overall performance on both verbal and nonverbal tests. The verbal and performance IQ scores are derived by converting the raw scores to standard scores for each subtest and for each age range. The full scale IQ is derived by summing the obtained standard scores on all of the subtests. The resulting "three" IQ scores can be, and frequently are, somewhat different, since they are derived from performance on different types of tasks. When all other factors are equal, the full scale IQ is used as the best general estimate of intellectual functioning. However, the distinction between a verbal IQ and a performance IQ has made the WAIS a relatively popular test among clinicians, especially for clients like deaf persons, whose intelligence might be grossly underestimated if it were derived from tasks which require verbal skills. Indeed, many authors, e.g., Vernon and Brown (1964), feel that the performance subtests of the Wechsler scales are the most appropriate measure of IQ for the deaf. Reliability and validity estimates for the performance scales of the Wechsler tests have been found to be acceptable (Brill, 1962; Evans, 1966; Pickles, 1966), although these estimates are somewhat lower for deaf persons than for the general population.

Wechsler has also developed the Wechsler Intelligence Scale for Children (WISC) and the Wechsler Preschool and Primary Scale of Intelligence (WPPSI), which also yield verbal, performance, and full scale IQ scores. All of the Wechsler scales have been comparatively well standardized. Test manuals are available giving detailed instructions for their administration and scoring, and norms from relatively large, representative samples of the U. S. population are available for evaluating specific scores. Wechsler's IQ is also a deviation IQ, that is, raw scores are transformed into standard scores with a mean of 100 and a standard deviation of 15. The WISC has recently been revised in 1974 (known as the WISC-R). Although some of the items have been changed, and the norms have been brought up to date with a better sampling of minorities, the overall format remains the same as described above.

A recent survey of testing practices with deaf children (Levine, 1974) indicated that the Wechsler scales are clearly a favorite among psychologists for evaluating the intelligence of deaf school age children and adolescents. Other tests of intelligence used with some frequency were the Leiter, the Hiskey-Nebraska, the Goodenough-Harris, the Arthur Adaptation of the Leiter, the Columbia Mental Maturity, the Merrill-Palmer Scale, Ravens' Progressive Matrices, and the Peabody Picture Vocabulary Test.

All published tests of intelligence share certain properties which are required for minimal levels of reliability and validity. These are fundamental requirements of such tests. Reliability refers to repeatability. A reliable test is one which can be trusted to yield the same or at least a very similar score at a later date or in a different testing situation. Validity refers to the ability of a test to measure what it is supposed to measure and to predict fairly accurately what it is supposed to predict. Some tests measure up to appropriate standards for reliability and validity better than others. Specialists in testing are accustomed to reading the accompanying literature on a test very carefully and to looking up reviews of the test in question in one of the Buros publications (for example, Buros, 1972).

Among the assumptions which must be met by an intelligence test and its administration are the following:

1. The knowledge which is required for a successful performance must be generally available to the individual who is being tested without any need for special training or instruction. If the item tests something that is taught specifically in school, then the item introduces a bias against those who happened to be educated differently. This principle of intelligence test construction implies that the test items should not discriminate against the persons being tested by reflecting a racial, ethnic, religious, or any known kind of cultural bias.

2. Sufficient information should be available on the performance that is typical of the population to which the person being tested belongs, so that his performance can be evaluated relative to the population. Such data are generally called the test's norms, and the normative data constitute an important aspect of a test's standardization. Normative data should be available from all of the populations from which individuals might be drawn for testing.

3. The test manual should provide clear information regarding both the administration and the scoring of the test. This is a second aspect of a test's standardization. It ensures that all subjects are tested in the same manner, no matter who does the testing. It also ensures that all responses will be scored similarly, no matter who does the scoring. Any departure from standard procedures for administering or scoring a test, however slight, renders invalid the norms which are ordinarily used to evaluate the resulting scores.

4. It is assumed that the test administrator is able to conduct the examination correctly and efficiently and that he or she is able to establish appropriate rapport with the client. This implies that the examiner is able to communicate comfortably with the client not only at the level of ensuring that the instructions were correctly understood but also, at a more personal level, of ensuring that the client is properly motivated to do his best on the tasks.

5. It is assumed that the outcome of the assessment, the score, is subject to a certain amount of error. The same test administered at a different time in a different place by a different examiner is likely to yield slightly different results. The most that can be said about an obtained score is that it identifies a range within which the true score is likely to fall given that all of the previous assumptions (1 through 4) have been met. This point is often overlooked or misunderstood by individuals not familiar with the principles of test construction. For example, if a client obtains an IQ score

of 101 on the first administration and a score of 97 on a second admini-stration, this might be misinterpreted as representing a change from above average to below average. This is simply not the case, as both scores should be interpreted as within the average range. In reality, there is no difference between the two scores, since random variations of that large an amount would be expected by chance.

TESTING DEAF CLIENTS

Under most circumstances, it is difficult to demonstrate that the necessary assumptions have been met for administering intelligence tests to deaf persons and for interpreting the results in the usual manner. The first assumption, that the information is equally available to all persons tested, is clearly violated for minority groups for whom English may be a second language and who did not attend regular public schools. In addition, to the extent that the deaf person's affiliation with the deaf linguistic community introduces him to social structures, values, and institutions that diverge more or less from those of the larger society, intelligence tests that have been standardized on the larger society are likely to discriminate against deaf persons. Deaf persons do not have equal access to culturally bound information or understandings which are likely to be explicitly or implic-itly required by the test. If important decisions affecting the tested person's welfare are based on his performance on a test which discrimi-nates against him because of a cultural bias, he has a right to seek relief through court action.

The second assumption, that norms are available against which the performances of individuals can be evaluated, can be questioned as well. For most of the tests that are presently being used with deaf school age children (Levine, 1974), deaf norms are not available, and deaf persons were not represented in the original sample on which the tests were standardized. The only major exception to this statement is the Hiskey-Nebraska test; both deaf and hearing norms are available. But they have not been revised lately, and the Hiskey-Nebraska test does not compare favorably with tests like the WISC on other counts, such as standardization and intercorrelations among the subtests.

The need for appropriate norms, however, is a complex issue. There are grounds for arguing that separate norms for deaf populations are not desirable, since they might foster paternalistic and discriminatory practices which are detrimental to appropriate educational treatment. Moreover, if the purpose of the testing is to predict how the individual will function in the larger society, the test might prove to have good predictive validity even though the norms might have limited utility on other counts. In fact, as the American Psychological Association (1974) monograph on standards points out, "It is incorrect to use the unqualified phrase, 'the validity of the test.' *No test is valid for all purposes or in all situations or for all groups of individuals*" (p. 31). The validity of a test must always be related to the use to which its results are put. Consequently, generating deaf norms for an intelligence test, while desirable for providing certain information which might be useful, will not by itself ensure that the test results will, then, be correctly interpreted. Nevertheless, the most frequent complaint volunteered by the respondents to Levine's (1974) questionnaire was the lack of appropriate instruments and the absence of appropriate norms, resulting in problems relating both to the selection and administration of tests and to the interpretation of the results. Individuals who know what norms are for obviously wish they had them.

The third assumption, calling for standardized procedures for administering and scoring the tests, is also clearly violated in most testing of deaf clients. Instructions on most intelligence tests are given verbally, and it is assumed that the client has sufficient hearing to be able to understand them. This assumption can obviously be questioned when the client is deaf. As a result, a number of modifications of the commonly used IQ test have been made so that the instructions can be given nonverbally. The reader interested in detailed descriptions of these modifications is referred to Reed (1970) and Sattler (1974). There are, however, two basic problems with these modifications. First, they require a good deal of additional skill and practice to be able to administer them successfully. Second, and more importantly, the use of nonverbal instructions is a significant violation of the standardized procedures upon which the norms and predictive validity of the test were based, as they were derived for the test when verbal instructions were used. We simply do not know whether the use of nonverbal instructions would facilitate, interfere with, or not affect the performance of individuals with normal hearing, nor whether performance would then still relate to the same degree with intelligence as when the standard administration procedures are used. It can be argued, similarly, that any sign language interpretation of the instructions would also violate the standardization procedures and make comparisons with the norms tenuous at best. The advantages of these modifications lie in their ability to determine whether there are some conditions under which the client can perform the task and, perhaps, related tasks. While such information has practical value, the resulting violations of the standardized procedures potentially reduce the value of the information obtained on intellectual functioning. There is no solution to this dilemma.

The fourth assumption, that the examiner be able to communicate comfortably with the client and establish sufficient rapport to be sure that the instructions are understood and that the client is well motivated, is, in practice, very difficult to meet. For deaf persons whose first language is Sign, communication in their preferred mode would violate the principle of standardized procedures mentioned previously. In any case, Levine's survey (1974), which was addressed to specialists serving deaf clients, revealed that half the respondents could not communicate manually, and three-fourths of the remainder rated their own sign language skills as fair to poor. However, the majority of the respondents' clients used manual methods to communicate, either alone or in combination with oral methods. The situation is not a promising one, since there are no training facilities where psychologists are being prepared in large numbers for serving deaf clients. Eighty-three percent of Levine's respondents reported on-the-job experience as their only preparation for dealing with deaf clients. Moreover, 90% of the respondents spent less than half of their work load with deaf clients, suggesting that their on-the-job experience was less than optimal for developing a high level of competence. The professional training of the respondents was mixed; only 16 of the 162 respondents reporting their degree qualifications had a doctoral degree. Nine reported a bachelor's degree as the highest degree earned. Three reported "certificates of specialization." The remainder had a master's degree as their terminal degree. It is painfully clear that a cadre of well-trained, professionally competent psychologists, who are able to communicate comfortably with deaf clients both orally and manually, simply does not exist.

If it could be assumed that deaf children are as highly motivated as typical white, middle class Americans to perform well on standardized tests, some of the difficulties associated with marginally competent personnel might be mitigated. Unfortunately, the opposite is the case. Deaf children are given little incentive to outperform one another or to earn the highest possible score on intelligence tests. They are generally unaware of the extent to which a high score might give them benefits which they would subsequently experience. Tests which stress speed or sustained concentrated effort are likely to be treated with some diffidence by many deaf persons. It should be mentioned, of course, that a high score on a demanding test is more trustworthy and potentially more valid than a low one, since it is difficult to imagine how a deaf person could do better than "he was able." But a low score must always be viewed with considerable suspicion, since there are many reasons other than lack of competence which might account for it.

Finally, the fifth assumption, that all tests are subject to a certain amount of measurement error, potentially may play a greater role in the assessment of deaf clients than in persons with normal hearing. It should be recalled that measurement error refers to the influence of all of the factors which affect test scores, but which are not directly related to what is being measured, which is intelligence in the present case. Typically, a statistical estimate of the amount of error expected from these sources is available in the test manual. Of course, this estimate is based on the population on which the test was standardized and, probably, did not include deaf persons. As indicated earlier, many of the sources of measurement error, such as rapport, comprehension of instructions, motivation to compete, etc., might be expected to have a relatively greater influence on the scores obtained by deaf clients. Indeed, one might expect both the number of sources of measurement error and the magnitude of their influence to result in a far larger measurement error for deaf persons than that reported in the test manual.

As can be seen, with deaf clients one can readily question each of the basic assumptions which are necessary for a reasonable derivation and interpretation of the IQ score. The scores obtained when these assumptions are violated can be considered no more than crude estimates of intellectual functioning. Often they may be very misleading. Although some of the information obtained from IQ test performance might have some potential practical value, it is doubtful that an IQ score by itself will adequately reflect the intellectual development of the deaf. Before discussing how one might integrate the information from the IQ score with other types of information in order to make some practical judgments and predictions, it is important to consider other ways in which intellectual development has been investigated.

OTHER STANDARDIZED TESTS

Given the precautions recommended for interpreting the results of intelligence tests, it is reasonable to inquire whether the results of other kinds of standardized tests, such as achievement tests or aptitude tests, might yield useful information. As with intelligence tests, the answer is yes, but only if equally strict safeguards are kept in mind.

Owing largely to the efforts of the Office of Demographic Studies at Gallaudet College in Washington, D.C., a considerable body of information is available on the results of annual administrations of Stanford Achievement Tests in schools and classes for deaf children. These data are published in the form of monographs which summarize the results and discuss the precautions that are appropriate for interpreting them. One of these monographs (DiFrancesca, 1972) presents tables of grade levels achieved by deaf pupils from below 6 years of age to 21 and over on the various forms of the 1964 edition of the Stanford Achievement Test Battery (Primary I, Primary II, Intermediate I, Intermediate II, and Advanced). Table 1 reveals that the only substantial "gains" occurred as the pupils were shifted from a lower to a higher form of the test and, therefore, to a higher floor. (The floor of a test is the lowest score that would be expected by chance.)

Since this is a rather strong claim to make about the performances of deaf children, illustrative data from the DiFrancesca (1972) monograph are presented in Table 1. The results are for the Arithmetic Battery, and they are limited to children who were profoundly deaf (hearing threshold levels reported as 99 dB and above). A similar table can be found in Furth (1973) for paragraph meaning scores reported in a previous monograph (Gentile and DiFrancesca, 1969). Two features of Table 1 warrant special attention. First, it is clear that there is very little improvement with age

Table 1. Mean grade equivalents of profoundly deaf children on the total arithmetic battery of the 1964 edition of the Stanford Achievement Test[a]

Ages in years	Battery				
	Primary I	Primary II	Intermediate I	Intermediate II	Advanced
6	1.4 (71)[b]				
7	1.5 (96)				
8	1.6 (149)	2.4 (15)			
9	1.8 (193)	2.8 (60)			
10	1.8 (219)	3.1 (126)			
11	1.8 (208)	3.2 (202)			
12	1.8 (246)	3.5 (264)	4.6 (43)		
13	1.9 (113)	3.8 (210)	5.2 (66)	6.0 (15)	
14	1.8 (106)	3.9 (191)	5.1 (85)	6.5 (18)	
15	1.9 (64)	4.2 (163)	5.4 (116)	6.7 (47)	8.1 (15)
16	1.8 (50)	4.3 (132)	5.2 (101)	6.7 (48)	7.9 (34)
17	1.9 (37)	4.1 (102)	5.4 (96)	6.5 (56)	8.5 (45)
18	1.8 (25)	4.4 (91)	5.6 (86)	6.5 (60)	8.4 (40)
19	1.7 (17)	4.4 (48)	5.7 (70)	7.1 (47)	8.6 (24)
20		4.2 (18)	5.3 (34)	7.2 (22)	7.9 (9)

[a]The data in this table are taken from publication D-9 of the Office of Demographic Studies and are used here with the permission of the director, Dr. Raymond J. Trybus.
[b]Numbers in parentheses refer to number of Ss.

within the same form of the test. From age 6 to age 19, the grade level goes from 1.4 to 1.7 on Primary I, and from age 8 to age 20 the grade level goes from 2.4 to 4.2 on Primary II. The situation is no more impressive for the more advanced forms. On Intermediate I the improvement is from 4.6 at age 12 to 5.3 at age 20, and on Intermediate II it is from 6.0 at age 13 to 7.2 at age 20. On the Advanced form, performance ranged from a low of 7.9 to a high of 8.6.

A second feature of Table 1 deserving attention is that over 400 teenagers were given the Primary I form of the battery. In fact, of the 2,500 deaf pupils 13 years old and older whose performances are reported in Table 1, 54% were given either Primary I or Primary II. This indicates a clear judgment on the part of responsible educators that there was something improper about choosing a test form for deaf children on the basis of their chronological age. Whether it was proper to administer a different form, one prescribed for much younger children, is open to question, but it was obviously considered to be the lesser of evils by persons who are presently responsible for testing deaf children. Only 19% of the pupils over 12 years of age who are represented in Table 1 were administered the Intermediate II or the Advanced form of the test.

Does this all mean that deaf children are learning nothing in school? We think not. We do think, however, that what they are learning is not being measured by standard achievement tests. Achievement tests were designed to measure what children learn in a formal educational program. Since the course of study for deaf children often does not correspond with the typical curricula for hearing children, especially in the higher grades, it is questionable whether an achievement test designed for all public school children is at all appropriate for deaf children. We believe that a rather clear case can be made for developing special achievement tests for deaf children with deaf norms and with appropriate procedures for administering them. A step in this direction is now being made by the Office of Demographic Studies. A special edition of the 1973 Stanford Achievement Test is in preparation for use among hearing-impaired children. Whether a revision of an existing instrument is the appropriate solution to the present problem or whether an entirely new instrument will need to be developed can be answered only on the basis of experience.

As with IQ tests, deaf children's English language deficiencies are a major problem for testing. Tests using English language instructions, comprised of items presented in English prose, and requiring a response to alternatives presented in English might well elicit substandard performances. Indeed, the same issues and problems that were examined in limiting the value of IQ scores as measures of intellectual development can be raised in questioning the value of current standard achievement test scores as measures of what deaf children have learned in school. If schools for deaf children wish to base decisions on what the child has learned, they clearly need achievement tests that are demonstrably more valid for this purpose than existing instruments, and they need procedures for administering them that are likely to give deaf children a fair opportunity to demonstrate their various competencies. This issue is made somewhat pressing as recent interest in mainstreaming has raised questions as to how deaf children may be judged "ready" for placement in a regular classroom. If standardized achievement test results are to be used to determine an appropriate grade placement for deaf children, it will become increasingly important to determine how high a score relative to normal grade level achievement is "good enough," and to determine how much of a disparity in chronological age is to be tolerated for the sake of placing deaf children with hearing children who appear to be functioning at the same grade levels. Given the current state of the art, it is clearly hazardous to rely heavily on grade level scores obtained from administrations of a standard achievement test battery.

We hasten to add that we believe that educators who are responsible for training deaf pupils appear to be quite aware of the doubtful validity of the results of standardized tests that they may be using. We see no evidence that teachers are prone to believe a single test battery's results when the results do not agree with what the teachers know to be true of their pupils from other observations of their ability. More than once, supervising teachers and principals have asked us how we could interpret standardized achievement test results obtained from their pupils, implying that they were uncertain as to how much confidence they should place in them. Our answer has been uniformly, "Very cautiously." Thus, the use of IQ and standard achievement test scores by themselves as the sole measures of deaf children's intellectual development and learning would appear to be limited.

EXPERIMENTAL STUDIES

There is another source of information on deaf children's intellectual development derived from a tradition in psychology that is somewhat separate from the interest in individual differences which gave rise to intelligence tests. This is the work of experimental psychologists who were interested in cognitive development.

Traditionally, deaf children's poor academic performance has been attributed to their language deficit. It is instructive that the term is often not qualified as an "English" language deficit, because the American Sign Language has not had, until very recently, any status in the eyes of linguists or educators as a language. Meanwhile, the widespread view that language is essential for rational thinking has influenced attitudes toward deafness, making it all the more important that "language" be taught to deaf children. "Every lesson is a language lesson" became a proverb in teacher training centers for specialists in deaf education.

The primacy of language over thinking has recently been vigorously challenged, and cognitive development is now perceived by many psychologists to be the basis rather than the result of specific linguistic achievements. A major impetus for the current cognitive revolution in psychology has come from the developmental theory of Jean Piaget (1950). The application of Piaget's theory to a psychology of deafness implied that deaf children could learn to think logically without relying on competence in a conventional language system (Furth, 1966). A survey of deaf children's performances on a wide variety of tasks assessing rule learning, use of logical symbols, Piaget-type tasks, memory, and perception (Furth, 1971) revealed that, in spite of a general linguistic deficiency, deaf children often performed as well as their hearing age peers, and implied that language is not a necessary condition for success on these tasks. Moreover, deaf children who had shown a developmental lag on these tasks relative to hearing children at younger ages sometimes "caught up" at older ages, even though their language development was still lagging far behind the levels of competence found in their peers with normal hearing. On the basis of these results, Furth concluded that a general experiential deficit is a far more defensible explanation than their proverbial language deficit for the developmental lags that deaf children sometimes manifest on cognitive tasks. Furth (1973) saw the same kind of parallel between deaf children and children growing up in rural Appalachia that Schlesinger and Meadow (1972) have seen between deaf children and children who are the victims of discrimination because of race or social class. In other words, these authors are suggesting that performance deficits of deaf children result from a lack of appropriate experience or opportunity rather than from differences in native ability.

Evidence is accumulating that, in spite of interesting and important differences between visual and auditory processing of information gained through experience, the central processes of learning, memory, perception, and cognition in deaf and hearing persons are functionally similar. For example, when given a Sign Association Test patterned after the familiar Word Association Tests, deaf children show the same developmental tendency to volunteer an association from the same part of speech as the stimulus word (or Sign) that is characteristic of hearing children (Tweney and Hoemann, 1973). Deaf adolescents not only organize their knowledge of English words in semantic categories that are similar to the semantic categories used by hearing adolescents, but they also reveal a similar hierarchical structure in their subjective lexicon (Tweney, Hoemann, and Andrews, 1975). School age deaf children show both the same relative effects of proactive interference in short-term memory and the same release from interference that is predicted by theories of memory which suggest that material is encoded categorically (Hoemann, Andrews, and DeRosa, 1974). Taken together, these studies indicate that deaf children and young adults manifest an adaptive tendency to understand their world in terms of conceptual categories, which provide a basis both for organizing their linguistic symbols and for storing and retrieving information from memory. All of this is accomplished, of course, without acoustic mediators and without the kinds of mnemonic or attentional aids that are usually available to persons who have normal access to a conventional language system.

This is not to suggest that deaf children's performances in cognitive tasks are uniformly satisfactory. They often lag the performance levels of hearing children by several years. Inadequate rehearsal strategies for memory tasks, inadequate incentive to perform at optimal levels in discovery tasks, and a general lack of experience or training in formal tasks of all kinds have all been advanced as possible explanations for the relatively poor performances of deaf children in tasks such as these. Moreover, the cognitive experimentalist shares many of the same problems as the clinician with regard to giving appropriate instructions, ensuring cooperation, and maintaining rapport in a task. For example, if an experimenter accepts an inappropriate response without comment so as not to influence subsequent responses, his acceptance may be interpreted by a deaf child as tacit approval. He may have inadvertently reinforced a response that was inappropriate, and, therefore, get more such responses. They will probably be interpreted as evidence of excessive perseveration on the part of the deaf child, when, in fact, it was the experimental procedures that were responsible for them. While data from experimental tasks have led to some exciting and constructive theorizing with regard to the intellectual development and functioning of deaf persons, they do not lend themselves well to simple explanations, and they often "illustrate that generalizations based on isolated studies are often premature" (Furth, 1971). Although much of the experimental work suggests that the cognitive processes and development of deaf persons follow a pattern similar to those of hearing persons, the same types of cautions suggested for IQ and achievement tests must be exercised with these results. It remains difficult to determine whether differences in performance between deaf and hearing persons result from differences in cognitive or intellectual development or from factors unrelated to what is being measured, regardless of whether the measures are based on experimental tasks or on standardized tests.

CONCLUSIONS AND IMPLICATIONS:
ASSESSMENT OF GENERAL COMPETENCE

By this time, the reader is aware that it is relatively difficult to assess adequately the intellectual development of deaf persons. The purpose of the previous discussion was to clarify the reasons for this difficulty. But even when rehabilitation counselors have no illusions about the realities of the situation, they are still in a position which requires them to make judgments, decisions, and recommendations based on the information that is available to them at the time. A logical question to ask is how to make maximum use of this available information while, at the same time, avoiding the types of misinterpretations discussed throughout this chapter.

Part of the answer to this question involves having a clear knowledge of specifically what one is trying to predict or to determine from this information. For example, if one is attempting to determine how well a client will function in a situation with particular sets of demands, such as an assembly line job with infrequent supervision, then the best predictor would be the client's previous performance on similar tasks with similar supervisory conditions. In general, if one is trying to predict competency in a new situation, then the best indicators are competencies in previous situations with similar characteristics. This relationship is a reasonably good rule regardless of what the specific new situation happens to be. Examples would include: predicting who is likely to benefit from a particular training program, how well an individual will function on a job, what counseling strategy is likely to "reach" the client, etc. In this sense, measures of intellectual development and academic achievement can be considered good predictors of relative success in those situations in which the skills necessary are similar to those being assessed by these measures.

It is not surprising, therefore, that, although far from perfect, IQ and achievement test scores tend to be reasonably good predictors of success in a wide variety of situations for the general population with normal hearing. As might be expected, however, these scores tend to be woefully inadequate predictors of relative success for the majority of the deaf population. In order to improve upon this picture, it is necessary to put these obtained scores in perspective and to view them as only one estimate of the general competence of the individual. There are many ways in which a person can display general competence, which may be defined as the ability to successfully function and adapt to the demands of the environment.

Therefore, we propose that an evaluation of the intellectual development of deaf persons be based on as broad a spectrum of their adaptive behaviors as possible within the limitations of time and resources available. Specifically, we recommend that this broad spectrum include the six areas of competence listed below. Armed with a knowledge of the client's functioning in these six areas, the rehabilitation counselor will hopefully be able not only to put the IQ score in proper perspective but also to obtain fruitful information upon which to base an estimate of the client's general competence. These six areas are as follows.

Social Competence

Social competence refers to the relative presence of age-appropriate interpersonal skills. Ideally, a knowledge of the client's social competence would include information on how well he relates to both peers and to authority figures, to persons with experience in working with the deaf and to persons without such experience. In general, the broader the range of social competence, the greater will be the number of situations in which the client can "get along." Conversely, inadequate or narrow social competence would be expected to limit the number of situations in which the client would function effectively.

Self Competence

Self competence refers to the client's relative confidence in his own abilities as well as to his awareness of his own strengths and weaknesses. It can be considered to include such concepts as self-esteem, self-worth, self-awareness, self-attitudes, etc. A knowledge of the client's self competence is important, since individuals who doubt their own competence are unlikely to convince others that they are competent in any area. Conversely, individuals with a strong and realistic self competence are not only likely to convince others of their potential abilities, but also, the belief, in itself, is likely to facilitate competence in other areas.

Physical Competence

Essentially physical competence refers to age-appropriate mastery of one's own body. It includes such things as dexterity, coordination, agility, mobility, etc. Strengths and weaknesses in this area of competence have direct implications for functioning in future situations.

Receptive Competence

Here we refer to the client's ability to comprehend and make use of information he receives from others, whether it be aurally (from speech) or visually (from reading, speechreading, or adjunctive, manual methods of communicating). It is also important to note whether the client's receptive competence is limited to those with experience in communicating with deaf persons or whether it extends to all individuals. Obviously, both the types of receptive competence and the numbers of individuals to whom the client can potentially demonstrate it are important factors in predicting adjustment to new situations. Specifically, the counselor needs to be aware of not only the client's receptive competence, but also the type and source of communication which the client will be asked to comprehend in order to make meaningful decisions about future functioning and/or training.

Expressive Competence

Expressive competence refers to the client's ability to communicate effectively to others. The key to the concept is the ability to make others understand what the client is attempting to convey, regardless of whether he transmits the message orally, manually, some combination of the two, or in writing. As with receptive competence, it is important to note both the types of expressive competence (oral, manual, written, or some combinations of them) and whether the recipient of the communication will need particular skills or training to fully comprehend it. Although expressive competence could be considered the "flip side" of receptive competence, it should be noted that competence in one of these areas does not automatically imply competence in the other. It is possible for an individual to demonstrate competence in only one, both, or neither of them as well as to display competence with different types of modalities and to different types of persons within each area. For example, the client may have expressive competence manually to those familiar with signing, but, at the same time, have receptive competence for both manual and oral communication regardless of the source. In this case, the client might be expected to function effectively in a wide variety of situations with a variety of people as long as there was no demand for him to express himself frequently to those unfamiliar with signing. Thus, it is quite possible for an individual to function effectively in some situations but not in others. This information is likely to be missed if one relied solely on a global measure, like an IQ score, as a predictor of effective functioning.

Adjustment Competence

Adjustment competence is a broad concept and includes such elements as the client's degree of acceptance of his handicap, a realistic awareness on his part of any potential limitations, and, most importantly, his ability to deal appropriately with the reactions of others to his handicap. The general public tends to have peculiar sets of responses to individuals with a handicap, like deafness. The client's awareness of these responses and his ability to deal with them effectively (as opposed to avoiding them) will greatly influence his functioning in many situations. While the other five areas of competence can be considered as applicable to all clients, this last one is of critical importance in making decisions with and for deaf clients. Difficulties in adjustment competence will require that both the client and the counselor make a decision on whether to consider counseling in this area to achieve competence or whether to acknowledge this difficulty and make appropriate plans to minimize its influence.

In general, the rehabilitation counselor can obtain a knowledge of the client's competence in each of these six areas through direct observation and/or through reports from others familiar with the client. We feel that knowledge of all six areas, as a necessary supplement to the IQ score, will be of considerable practical value in the decision-making process. With this practical focus, we are deliberately sidestepping the theoretical issue of whether competence in any one of these areas is any better a measure of intellectual development than the others or than an IQ score. Thus, we urge the counselor who needs practical information on the intellectual development of his client to use a variety of sources of information to make this estimate and, thereby, be in a better position to make rational and fair judgments, decisions, and recommendations.

REFERENCES

American Psychological Association. 1974. Standards for Educational and Psychological Tests. American Psychological Association, Washington, D.C.

Brill, R. G. 1962. The relationship of Wechsler IQs to academic achievement among deaf students. Except. Child., 28:315–321.

Buros, O. K. (ed.). 1972. Mental Measurement Yearbook. 7th Ed. Gryphon Press, Highland Park, N.J.

DiFrancesca, S. 1972. Academic Achievement Test Results of a National Testing Program for Hearing Impaired Students: United States, Spring

1971. Office of Demographic Studies, Gallaudet College, Washington, D.C.

Evans, L. 1966. A comparative study of the Wechsler Intelligence Scale for Children (Performance) and Raven's Progressive Matrices with deaf children. Teacher of the Deaf 64:76–82.

Furth, H. G. 1966. Thinking without Language: Psychological Implications of Deafness. Free Press, New York.

Furth, H. G. 1973. Deafness and Learning: A Psychosocial Approach. Wadsworth, Belmont, Calif.

Gentile, A., and S. DiFrancesca. 1969. Academic Achievement Test Performance of Hearing Impaired Students. Gallaudet College Press, Washington, D. C.

Hoemann, H. W., C. E. Andrews, and D. V. DeRosa. 1974. Categorical encoding in short-term memory by deaf and hearing children. J. Speech Hear. Res. 17:426–431.

Levine, E. 1974. Psychological tests and practices with the deaf: A survey of the state of the art. Volta Rev. 76:298–319.

Myerson, L. 1963. A psychology of impaired hearing. In W. M. Cruickshank (ed.), Psychology of Exceptional Children and Youth 2nd ed., pp. 118–191. Prentice-Hall, 1962. Englewood Cliffs, N.J.

Piaget, J. 1950. The Psychology of Intelligence. Harcourt, Brace & World, New York.

Pickles, D. G. 1966. The Wechsler Performance Scale and its relationship to speech and educational response in deaf slow-learning children. Teacher of the Deaf 64:382–392.

Reed, M. 1970. Deaf and partially hearing children. In P. Mittler (ed.), The Psychological Assessment of Mental and Physical Handicaps, pp. 403–441. Methuen, London.

Sattler, J. M. 1974. Assessment of Children's Intelligence. W. B. Saunders Company, Philadelphia.

Schlesinger, H. S., and K. P. Meadow. 1972. Sound and Sign: Childhood Deafness and Mental Health. University of California Press, Berkeley, Calif.

Tweney, R. D., and H. W. Hoemann. 1973. The development of semantic associations in profoundly deaf children. J. Speech Hear. Res. 16:309–318.

Tweney, R. D., H. W. Hoemann, and C. E. Andrews. 1975. Semantic organization in deaf and hearing subjects. J. Psycholing. Res. 4:61–73.

Vernon, M., and D. W. Brown. 1964. A guide to psychological tests and testing procedures in the evaluation of deaf and hard-of-hearing children. J. Speech Hear. Disord. 29:414–422.

Personality
and Social Development
of Deaf Persons

KATHRYN P. MEADOW

Most theories of personality and social development stress the importance of the individual's early experiences in helping to shape his behavior and his life adjustment. In the sense that many deaf people share a number of early life experiences, we might expect that they may share some common problems and some common ways of coping with the environment. In this sense, it can be useful to consider the personality and social development of deaf persons in general terms. However, it is useful to talk in general terms only if appropriate caution is taken that damaging stereotypes are not formulated from overgeneralizations. There is as wide a range of personality patterns among deaf persons as there is among persons with normal hearing. Although it is convenient to talk about personality patterns and social development "of deaf persons," there are many subgroups within the general category of the hearing impaired. Some of the subgroups of deaf people are based on the social or the demographic indicators that divide the general population: sex, age, race, and social class. Additional classifications that reflect different social experiences or different social adaptations for deaf people include: degree of hearing loss,

Support from Maternal and Child Health (Grant MC-R-060160-05-0) and from the Office of Education, Bureau for the Education of the Handicapped (Grant OEG-0-75-1441) made much of this work possible. Portions of this material will appear in *Deafness and Child Development,* to be published by the University of California Press.

age at onset of deafness, etiology of hearing loss, hearing status of family members, type of schooling, preferred communication mode, and degree of identification with the deaf subculture. Understanding of a particular deaf client requires knowledge about all or most of these factors.

It is both convenient and meaningful to limit our definition of deafness to a hearing loss so profound as to preclude the understanding of speech and one that predated the acquisition of language. Thus, the primary handicap of deafness is the limitation of communication, in the same sense that the primary handicap of blindness is the limitation of mobility. Deafness is an exceedingly complex disability. It incorporates elements of medical, audiological, linguistic, sociological, and psychological factors that influence the developmental process and that contribute to some of the experiences that deaf children often share. It is these shared experiences rather than the hearing deficit itself that lead us to talk about a "psychology of deafness." At least some of the noxious experiences shared by deaf persons are subject to change. Therefore, some of the apparently shared personality characteristics are not a necessary accompaniment of a hearing handicap.

Two major categories of shared early experiences are particularly important in the personality and social development of the deaf. First is the fact that communication between most deaf children and their parents is either absent or very rudimentary during the important early years of the child's life. These are the years when parents and children would ordinarily have the most constant and exclusive contact with each other. The second important major category of early life experience shared by deaf persons is the usual response of parents to the diagnosis of a hearing handicap in a young child. This early response is the first of a long series of social responses to handicap with which handicapped persons must cope. Parents, however, often respond to diagnosis with sorrow, shock, shame, guilt, and anger. Their attitudes about the meaning of deafness influence their treatment of the deaf child, thus influencing the child's personality and social development.

SOCIAL DEVELOPMENT

Social and Emotional Maturity

The most frequently stated generalization about the psychological and social development of deaf individuals is that they seem to exhibit a high degree of "emotional immaturity." Levine (1956) has described this complex in terms of "egocentricity, easy irritability, impulsiveness, and suggestibility." Myklebust (1960) found that deaf persons were immature in "caring for others." Altshuler (1974) characterized deaf patients as demonstrating "egocentricity, a lack of empathy, dependency." The term "maturity" in a social sense often refers to an individual's ability to care for himself, to accept responsibility for his actions and his destiny, and to be independent. The Vineland Social Maturity Scale was designed to measure children's capacity to care for themselves and to engage in activities that lead to ultimate independence. It measures abilities in self-help, self-direction, locomotion, occupation, communication, and social relations.

A large number of studies of deaf children has been reported showing that deaf children received lower scores on the Vineland Scale of Social Maturity than did hearing children of comparable ages. One study was done with parents and children with a variety of handicaps, including deafness. All the handicapped children were found to be deficient in self-help skills. However, the more remarkable aspect of the report was the discrepancy between the tasks that the children were *capable* of performing and those that they actually did for themselves. This suggests that parents generalize from the narrow range of tasks that a handicapped child actually cannot do and assume that there is a much larger spectrum of tasks of which he is incapable. Eventually, the assumed inability becomes a real inability because the child does not have the opportunity to practice tasks and develop new levels of expertise. In addition, it takes more patience and time for handicapped children to perform the trial-and-error process of skill acquisition—time and patience that parents may not have or be unwilling to give. For deaf children with deficient communication skills, it takes additional time and patience merely to communicate what is expected, required, and necessary for the performance of even a simple task.

Human development is a cumulative process. That is, readiness for the development of one age-appropriate skill is based on the development of another skill at an earlier age. By the same token, deficiencies in tasks requiring self-responsibility and maturity may be cumulative as well. Parents and other caretakers who observe that a child or adolescent is unable to perform one kind of self-help task may be even more reluctant to demand or to allow him to perform another kind of task that is appropriate for the next age level.

Many deaf children and adolescents are educated in state residential schools. (The National Census of the Deaf Population showed that one-half of deaf persons aged 25–64 in 1972 had been educated *exclusively* in residential schools.) Residential living influences the development of maturity, although most administrators today are aware of these factors and attempt to create an environment that encourages independence. Some of the disadvantages of the residential setting stem from the nature of dormitory life and the administrative hazards inherent in large institutions. When children live together in groups, it is necessary that rules be made that can be applied to the group, sometimes conflicting with needs of individual children. Chores that might be assigned to children in their family settings may be performed by maintenance personnel in an institution. Opportunities for privacy and space for private activities are less frequent in a residential school than in a home. When students reach the age when boy-girl relationships begin to be explored, both parents and school personnel become anxious about the possible consequences of sexual activities. This leads to restrictive rules and fewer opportunities for the development of relationships than might be found in the family environment of other adolescents. Thus, the limited social opportunities of the deaf adolescent in the residential school can add to an already underdeveloped sense of self-responsibility and social immaturity.

One research study conducted with deaf students in a residential school compared those whose parents were deaf to another group in the same school whose parents had normal hearing. These students were rated by their teachers and counselors on several dimensions of social and personal development. The students with deaf parents received consistently higher or more positive ratings for "maturity," "responsibility," and for "independence." The students with deaf parents had all experienced early family communication since the parents ordinarily used American Sign language with them from infancy onward. In addition, the reactions of the deaf parents to the diagnosis of deafness in their child were considerably less traumatic than that experienced by hearing parents. (It should be noted that no more than 10% of deaf children have both a deaf mother and a deaf father.)

Many of the traits that have been used to characterize deaf persons might also be used to describe a person who is thought to be "immature." Three traits that have been used again and again are "impulsivity," "egocentricity," and "rigidity." If we look at the meaning, or at the behavioral patterns that these trait descriptors are intended to summarize, it is not difficult to speculate that these characteristics develop readily among any group where early communication was absent or imperfect.

Impulsiveness refers to behavior that is not based on careful, coherent, advance planning. The impulsive person may be unable to plan a course of action and adhere to it. He may make rash choices based on a desire for immediate gratification rather than on the expectation of long-term gains. Building long-term goals may require an ability to think out or to imagine (or to live in fantasy) future possibilities that stem from one or another present decision. If we look to the early experiences of deaf children, we see that language is important for the expression of time. Those who do not have language are restricted by the tyranny of the present in terms of both time and space. Parents can communicate in a rudimentary way to their deaf children about things that are present in the same room or about events that are current. Language is necessary if one wishes to communicate about events that occurred in the past or that will take place in the future. Thus, deaf children often have not had the experience of communicating about future plans or reminiscing about memories from the past. Most parents, when they want their child to wait to receive a particular treat or experience, are able to tell him when he can expect to receive the desired object and why the delay is necessary. Without language, this is difficult or impossible. Thus, parents of deaf children often yield to immediate demands or suffer temper tantrums that are uncomfortable for everyone. The deaf child does not learn easily to control his demands for immediate gratification by learning that sometimes he can expect to be given something at a later time.

Egocentricity describes a person whose world centers on or revolves around himself. A self-centered person is one who is unwilling or unable to consider the needs, the opinions, or the desires of others. He is unaware or uncaring about the effect of his behavior on other people. A part of the normal developmental process involves, first, the differentiation of oneself from others and, second, the realization that one's behavior affects the behavior of those around him in specific ways. Again, language or communication is important or perhaps even necessary if this process is to take place. One way in which a child becomes socialized to the ways of his society is through his desire to please his parents who communicate to him the norms of his particular group. Group norms are expressed in the person of the parent. Social approval or disapproval consists of parental approval or disapproval in the early years. If a child is to take into account the wishes of others, he must understand what it is about his behavior that affects significant others in either positive or negative ways. An explanation of emotions experienced by others is difficult without fairly complex language. The language of emotions is an area where deaf children are particularly deficient.

Rigidity refers to an inflexible approach to the world or to particular tasks. It reflects an inability to change one's demands or requests to conform to changing situations or events. It can also refer to a tendency to apply a once-learned rule indiscriminately. Thus, it is often said of deaf persons that they "live by the rule book of etiquette." It seems to be difficult for them to differentiate between the more and the less important situation for the application of a particular rule.

When deaf children are learning their first "rules" about acceptable and unacceptable ways of behaving, they may not learn the reasons surrounding a particular prohibition. The rule must be followed "because Mother says so," or "because Father will be angry." They do not have the benefit of learning explanations for the rules: "If you go too near the fire you will get burned"; "If you break my vase I will feel badly." Thus, rules are applied indiscriminately to new situations because the reasoning on which they are based is not understood. This indiscriminate application of rules then appears to be *rigidity*.

Deaf children seem to have particular difficulty in developing the idea of causality in both the physical world and the social world. The language of "why" and "because" does not come easily. It is hard to elicit a response to the question of "Why did you do such-and-such?" Hearing children at about age of 2 years threaten to drive their parents to the brink of insanity with incessant questions beginning with the word "why." Perhaps this stage of language is important for the incorporation of ideas of causality. A world that appears to be without rhyme or reason is more likely to be approached by means of a rigid set of rules.

Maturity: Implications for Rehabilitation Counselors

Vocational maturity is closely related to social and emotional maturity. It is more difficult to place an "immature" client on a job and to help him to remain on the job. The client who has been sheltered by his family and who has continued to be sheltered by his teachers is less likely to be ready to take responsibility on the job. For the deaf person, there is often a thin line between tasks that he can be expected to do for himself and tasks with which he needs some help because of his impaired hearing. In the same way that parents and teachers must tread this line in living and working with deaf children and adolescents, the rehabilitation counselor must tread the line in working with deaf adults. The rehabilitation counselor needs to foster independent behavior rather than reinforcing old patterns of dependency. Clients with long experience in surrendering their independence to others usually become skillful in demanding and maneuvering to continue their helplessness.

A prime example of issues around dependency of deaf clients centers on their realistic need for help in the use of the telephone. In making job applications and in setting up appointments for interviews with prospective employers, telephone contact obviously can save time and is usually more efficient. If the counselor is unaware of the trap of dependency and the long-term benefit to his client of increasing independence, he may make more telephone calls than are truly necessary. On the other hand, to insist that he will never make phone calls for deaf clients is a denial of the reality of the handicap.

Counselors can help deaf clients to become more mature by insisting that they find substitutes for direct telephone calls for changing or canceling appointments. This can become valuable experience for the kind of responsible behavior expected by employers for notification when absence from work is unavoidable. Helping a deaf client to make an on-going arrangement with a neighbor or to develop a signal system with the telephone can be very useful. Deaf adults can sometimes learn to use the telephone in limited ways with people whom they know, but often find this a frightening and threatening experience. The rehabilitation counselor who has developed a relationship with a deaf client may be able to help him deal with some fears in this area. The importance of keeping appointments and of being on time is something that immature persons— handicapped or not—often have difficulty in understanding.

Another hallmark—or even definition—of immaturity is the absence of many life experiences that are frequently assumed. Thus, we assume that any adult has had experience in using public transportation, in managing a budget of some kind, and in dealing with everyday bureaucracies encompassed in banks, medical services, and so forth. This is often not the case for persons who have led sheltered, dependent lives. The counselor may need to help some deaf clients with these basic experiential details before a successful job placement is possible. These kinds of considerations, all related to the relative maturity or immaturity of many deaf clients, lead to an important area for supervisors and administrators of rehabilitation services. One implication of the maturity level to be expected of deaf clients is that it often takes more counselor time to work with a caseload of hearing-impaired clients. To expect the same rate of successful job placements or to expect rehabilitation counselors for the deaf to carry the same caseload as specialists with other kinds of caseloads may be unrealistic. Some of the basic needs of deaf clients might be met as well, or perhaps even better, by a paraprofessional aide to the rehabilitation counselor. An aide who is deaf or who is fluent in sign language may be able to help in basic orientation that is prevocational in nature.

Finally, it is important to mention one more pitfall that is common for many helping professionals who work with deaf adolescents or young adults. This is the temptation to work with the client's parents rather than with the client himself. Often, parents are used to making decisions *for* their deaf children rather than *with* them or rather than encouraging them to make their decisions independently. Parents often present themselves to the rehabilitation counselor along with the young deaf adult, expecting to be totally involved in the decision-making process for training or for vocational planning. Counselors need to be prepared with tactful ways of encouraging the process of disengaging parents and their grown-up deaf children. This is another part of the definition of maturity.

Self-Image

The growth of self-image or identity goes hand in hand with social development. As a child begins to be an object to himself, as he sees himself reflected in the appraisals of others, he begins to understand both their behavior and his own. The child sees himself "mirrored" in the responses that important others make to him and gets a sense of his own worth from their reactions. Initially, a child's important others are his parents and his siblings. Gradually, his circle widens, and his self-image is affected by the responses of teachers, peers, storekeepers, and neighbors. Children who are handicapped begin to learn or to sense their difference very early. The positive or negative meaning attached to their definition of their "differentness" depends in large part on the feelings of significant others, particularly their parents. It is for this reason that parental responses to the diagnosis of deafness are so important to the development of the hearing-handicapped child. Parents who are ashamed or embarrassed about their child's deafness cannot help but communicate this to the child. He, in turn, incorporates their feelings about him, and they become a part of his self-image or self-concept.

The relative visibility of a handicap is important to the response that is evoked in others or to the stigma imposed on the handicapped person. Ironically, deafness itself is invisible; it is the means through which deaf persons *cope* with their handicap that make them visible. Thus, it is the hearing aid that gives one clue to the presence of a handicap; it is sign language that gives another clue to the presence of a handicap; unusual or distorted speech patterns that give a third clue. Parents who are not reconciled to their child's deafness may give subtle and ambiguous messages to him about his worth by giving ambiguous messages about his means of coping with his deafness. Sometimes parents do not want their deaf children to wear their hearing aids when they are photographed. Or they may remove the hearing aid when they put on the party dress or the Sunday suit. These incidents reflect parental attitudes that edge a child toward negative identity feelings in relation to his deafness.

For many years, the educational controversy about the means of communication to be used with deaf children was couched in terms of *either* sign/manual language *or* spoken/oral language. The dichotomy created by educators and adopted by parents meant that many deaf children were bound to be placed in an "identity bind" at some point in the lifespan. If spoken communication were the only acceptable communication and the deaf person's speech proved to be unintelligible for a majority of those he met, his identity became unacceptable to himself as it appeared to have been to his parents and teachers who insisted on speech only. If the deaf person learned sign language in adolescence, felt more comfortable using it for communication, and in relating to others who also used it, he might reject completely the use of hearing aids and speech that might serve to identify him with the nondeaf community.

Young deaf children rarely have the opportunity to meet deaf adults who might serve as positive role models for them. This means that some of them develop skewed ideas about their own identity and about their adult destinies. Some believe that they will develop hearing and speech as they grow older. Deaf teachers have been barred from teaching in most day schools and classes. Recently, as total communication became more acceptable, deaf teacher aides became assets in the classroom because of their fluent knowledge of sign language. In residential schools, where deaf people have found employment in the past, the kinds of jobs for which they could apply were limited. They usually were not hired to teach in the younger grades where instruction was probably by oral means only. Thus, they could teach in the upper grades or they could apply for jobs as dormitory counselors or houseparents. The status differential between teaching and dormitory staffs favored the teaching staff. Thus, the deaf students in residential schools saw their possible role models—that is, the other deaf persons in their environment—in the less desirable status positions.

The research comparing deaf students with deaf and with hearing parents also compared the self-image of the two groups. Students with deaf parents had significantly more positive scores on the self-image test than did the students with hearing parents. There were also some interesting differences in the children of deaf and hearing parents when different age groups were analyzed. Younger children of deaf parents had especially high levels of self-esteem; younger children of hearing parents had especially low levels of self-esteem. For older children, self-image scores were almost the same for the two groups with deaf and with hearing parents.

When day school students with hearing parents were tested later, their scores were almost identical to those of the residential students with hearing parents. Self-image was particularly low among those students whose hearing parents had high levels of educational achievement. This suggests that when deaf students feel that they are unable to fulfill their parents' expectations for them, they may have negative self-concepts.

Self-Image: Implications for Rehabilitation Counselors

Self-image, self-confidence, and positive self-concept are important to the job effectiveness of everyone. This area is even more important for the handicapped person, and for the deaf client no less than others. The single most critical way in which the image of the self for the deaf client is different than for others is the special link between communication mode and self-image. The phrase "my language is me" has special significance for deaf persons. By respecting the language or the preferred communication mode of the deaf client, two goals may be achieved: a positive sense of self is encouraged and rapport between counselor and client is established.

The important facet of this discussion is the necessity for the counselor to accept the client's *own* definition of preferred communication mode, rather than attempting to impose the counselor's definition of what is "best." This means that, ideally speaking, the rehabilitation counselor needs to be fluent in the entire range of possible communication modes that might be used by an individual client. These include: Ameslan, Signed English, "SEE signs," and oral English.

Ameslan refers to American Sign language. This is a gesture language with its own grammar and syntax and is used by most deaf adults who consider themselves to be members of the deaf subculture. Ameslan is, in fact, the major symbol of the cohesiveness of the in-group of the deaf community. For many deaf adults, acceptance of Ameslan is synonymous with acceptance of deafness. Thus, rehabilitation counselors of the deaf need to have some knowledge of sign language at the minimum. If they are not fluent, they need to learn and to have a skilled interpreter available when needed. One of the requests for service that is most likely to be made of counselors is the provision of an interpreter for legal, medical, or educational needs. Thus, they should be aware of interpreters who qualify for certification by the Registry of Interpreters for the Deaf in the particular area they serve.

Signed English approximates spoken English more closely than does Ameslan. It is the form of sign language that is utilized in the educational approach referred to as the "combined method" of speaking and signing simultaneously. However, it is like Ameslan in that verb tenses and noun modulations are not incorporated into the signed message. "SEE signs," on the other hand, do include these features in the signs as well as in the spoken portion of the communication. SEE signs are utilized in the educational approach that is being called "total communication." Total communication incorporates formal sign language, spoken language, and strict attention to amplification for deaf children both at home and in the classroom. More and more programs of deaf education are utilizing this approach at the present time. This means that the next generation or "cohort" of deaf students leaving schools will feel more at home with SEE signs, making it important for rehabilitation counselors to be fluent or at least aware and accepting of this form of communication as well. For 200 years, there has been bitter conflict among educators about the use of oral versus the use of manual communication with the deaf child. This conflict seems to be diminishing as the acceptance of total communication grows. A new controversy is brewing about the form that the sign language portion of total communication will take. While rehabilitation counselors may well form their own opinions about the educational issues, they need to accept their deaf clients' communication mode on an individual basis.

Some deaf clients will continue to rely exclusively on spoken communication with rehabilitation counselors. It takes the unfamiliar ear some time to learn and to become comfortable with deaf voices generally and with individual voices specifically. Use of paper and pencil or typewritten communication to help speed communication may be helpful. Often, young deaf adults who have grown up in strictly, or even militantly, oral environments welcome referrals to sign language classes. Even if they continue to use spoken communication as their preferred mode with the general community, familiarity with sign language can broaden their social horizons and sometimes make them more comfortable with their deaf identity. This is more likely to be true if the option is offered as a suggestion rather than as a prescription by the counselor.

Behavioral Problems of Deaf People

Deaf children are said to exhibit higher rates of behavior problems than comparable groups of children in the general population. Behavior problems have been described as of "epidemic proportions" among deaf children, with as many as 10 or 12% exhibiting severe emotional or behavioral disturbances. This is about five times the proportion that would be expected. The figures on which these estimates are based usually are collected from teachers of deaf students. Judgments are ordinarily made about the kinds of behavior that are most difficult to manage in a classroom. Thus, the aggressive, active, acting-out child is more likely to be identified than the shy, withdrawn child. An important consequence for the child of this kind of behavior is frequently exclusion from school. Since so many deaf children are considered problematic by their teachers, it is somewhat curious that the prevalence of severe mental illness is no

greater among deaf adults than is found in the general population. However, Rainer, Altshuler, and Kallmann (1969) suggested, on the basis of
their studies of the deaf population of New York State, that deaf adults
display more "problems of living." These show up as higher crime and
delinquency rates, higher rates of family and marital problems, and agency
referrals for problems of alcohol abuse or sexual acting-out.

The developmental basis for this array of problem behaviors is, of
course, diverse and varied. Many problems undoubtedly stem from frustration at the absence of communication, from family, school, and community response to handicap, and from negative self-image. Two other factors
must be mentioned, however. One is the high rate of physical and neurological handicaps in addition to deafness that is found among the current
generation of deaf children. Fully one-third of all deaf children have
another handicap in addition to their deafness. Secondly, the effect of
societal response to the kinds of behaviors that come to be labeled
"emotionally disturbed" often reinforces the very behavior patterns that
created difficulties in the first place. The child who is labeled a "bad boy"
is defined that way not only by others but also by himself. He then
becomes the "delinquent adolescent" and the "problem adult." Breaking
the cycle becomes more difficult at each developmental stage.

Behavior Problems: Implications for Rehabilitation Counselors

Deaf persons with additional problems of any kind are more difficult to
train, to place, and to counsel. When the additional problems take the
form of additional physical handicaps, however, solutions can take a more
specific form. If a solution takes the form of a mechanical device or a
technical innovation, it is less likely that human "failing" is responsible for
a breakdown in the counselor's planning. However, when a deaf client's
additional problems stem from behavior that is socially unacceptable or
that runs counter to institutional legal or administrative regulations, it is
more difficult to retain a nonjudgmental point of view. The rehabilitation
counselor's job is made harder with behaviorally difficult deaf persons
because of the paucity of institutions designed to care for them. There are
very few mental hospitals with wards where deaf patients can communicate with staff persons. There are few facilities for the treatment of deaf
alcoholics. There are almost no half-way houses that are able to provide
shelter for deaf patients. The rehabilitation counselor for the deaf needs
more access to mental health consultants. He needs to be able to refer deaf
clients for therapy with professionals who are skilled in various ways of
working with deaf patients. The relative absence of these facilities and of
training centers for mental health professionals who can work with the

deaf means that the rehabilitation counselor must often serve the difficult deaf client less well than he would like.

CONCLUSION

Perhaps the most important summary point to be made is the reiteration of a cautionary statement: deaf people are not all alike; there is as much variation among deaf people as there is among their hearing peers. The important facet of life experience that enables us to talk in terms of the "personality" or "psychology" of "the deaf" is the unfortunate shared factor of early language or communicative deficiencies. As more deaf children acquire language at the normal age and in an optimal, joyful family milieu, we can expect to see fewer deaf adults with the social-emotional problems and personality traits that stem from retarded language acquisition. An important implication of this picture is the need for rehabilitation workers to be concerned with the early experiences of their future deaf clients. Preventive rehabilitation may be more important for this group of handicapped persons than for any other. Early language has important implications for the whole person. The deaf person's communicative handicap cannot be entirely overcome in his adult years since early communicative deprivation has such profound consequences for personality and social development. For deaf persons, rehabilitation must begin in the cradle. Otherwise, the social and psychological consequences of the handicap are carried to the grave.

REFERENCES

Altshuler, K. Z. 1974. The social and psychological development of the deaf child: Problems, their treatment and prevention. Amer. Ann. Deaf. 119:365–376.

Garrett, J. F., and E. S. Levine. 1962. Psychological Practices with the Physically Disabled. Columbia University Press, New York.

Goffman, E. 1964. Stigma. Prentice-Hall, Inc., Englewood Cliffs, N.J.

Levine, E. S. 1956. Youth in a Soundless World, a Search for Personality. New York University Press, Washington Square, N. Y.

Meadow, K. P. 1975. The development of deaf children. In E. M. Hetherington, J. W. Hagen, R. Kron, and A. H. Stein (eds.), Review of Child Development Research, Vol. V, pp. 439–506. University of Chicago Press, Chicago.

Mindel, E. D., and M. Vernon. 1971. They Grow in Silence–The Deaf Child and His Family. National Association of the Deaf, Silver Spring, Maryland.

Myklebust, H. R. 1960. The Psychology of Deafness, Sensory Deprivation, Learning and Adjustment. Grune & Stratton, Inc., New York.

Rainer, J. D., K. Z. Altshuler, and F. J. Kallmann (eds.). 1969. Family and Mental Health Problems in a Deaf Population. 2nd Ed. Charles C Thomas, Springfield, Ill.

Schein, J. D. 1968. The Deaf Community: Studies in the Social Psychology of Deafness. Gallaudet College Press, Washington, D. C.

Schein, J. D., and M. T. Delk. 1974. The Deaf Population of the United States. National Association of the Deaf, Silver Spring, Maryland.

Schlesinger, H. S., and K. P. Meadow. 1972. Sound and Sign: Childhood Deafness and Mental Health. University of California Press, Berkeley, Calif.

Vernon, M. 1969. Sociological and psychological factors associated with hearing loss. J. Speech Hear. Res. 12:541–563.

5 | Vocational Development

ALAN LERMAN

Vocational adjustment of an individual has been seen by some as an isolated area of functioning, marginally influenced by personal history, personality attributes, and social development, governed by immediate factors such as the availability of jobs, acquired vocational skills, and the work environment. Alternatively, vocational adjustment is more frequently considered as current behavior related to general processes of individual growth and development which reflect themselves in what people choose and continue to do as careers.

THEORETICAL CONSIDERATIONS

Increasingly, it is assumed that choice and involvement in a career are the outgrowths of some process and are not accidental. With sufficient information about factors in a person's life that affect his choice and subsequent involvement, we might be able to understand and perhaps influence the course of vocational development.

It is true that, in many situations, environmental pressures place constraints on career choice and vocational adjustment. Poverty, prejudice, rigid societies, and institutions severely limit individual choices and restrict vocational development. Expanding, complex, and affluent societies offer greater flexibility and permit maximum individual development.

Individual studies relate vocational choice, satisfaction, career pattern, and success to antecedent behaviors or parallel behaviors. These have been reviewed by Super et al. (1957), Roe (1956), Hertzberg et al. (1957), and Borow (1964). While the results of these studies are often contradictory (which may be partly caused by differences in *samples,* as well as specific behaviors or characteristics studied, design, and methodological problems), the general impression is that this information lends support to the view that vocational behaviors are part of a process of vocational development.

Super and Overstreet (1960) appear to offer the most comprehensive theoretical framework for vocational development. Their model offers a sequence of life stages, together with a brief description of the nature of vocational behavior which seems accurate for each stage. The earliest phases of vocational development occur in the preadolescent period when the child views work and career in ways that are unrelated to reality factors. He considers adult roles in terms of fantasy, e.g., a fireman puts out fires and a policeman stops crime. His personal contacts and the information he receives through the media determine what he views as possible careers. In early adolescence, he explores his own abilities and extrapolates what he does well and what is considered socially useful or desirable to possible career choices. At the end of adolescence and in his early young adulthood, he still explores possible vocations with increasing concern to reality factors, e.g., schooling required, job opportunities, and actual financial rewards. For the next one or two decades, he works at establishing himself in a chosen occupation. Following this period, he directs his energies at maintaining his position and his level of functioning.

The basic principles for guiding development toward mature vocational functioning are: (1) behavior proceeds from random and undifferentiated activity to goal-directed specific activity; (2) that it is in the direction of increasing awareness and orientation to reality; and (3) that it goes from dependence to increasing independence.

MODEL OF VOCATIONAL DEVELOPMENT

Ideally, the goal of vocational rehabilitation is to assist the client in making a successful vocational adjustment, i.e., in securing a job which he performs competently and from which he receives some measure of satisfaction. Vocational adjustment itself is only one stage of an essentially two-stage process of vocational development. The first, the prevocational stage, consists of all behaviors associated with the world of work, short of actually seeking or obtaining employment. The second, the vocational stage, is concerned with all job-seeking behaviors and with actual vocational adjustment (job satisfaction and job satisfactoriness). Furthermore, the kinds of prevocational and vocational behaviors exhibited by a person are the result of certain individual and social factors. The selection of appropriate aspects of general individual functioning and general environmental influences, past or current, that may be considered relevant to vocational functioning is somewhat arbitrary. Since it is not possible to include the total life experiences, the selection is based on those aspects that appear to be the most directly related or have been shown to be related to prevocational or vocational behaviors. Those categories within the model are purposely left broad enough to permit the reader to select those aspects that he feels are most relevant. The relationship between these factors and behaviors is outlined in Figure 1.

In this scheme, true vocational behavior, including job-seeking and job adjustment, is determined by several internal and external factors. Internal factors governing the kinds of jobs the client will seek include the client's vocationally related traits, abilities, and interests, the extent of his knowl-

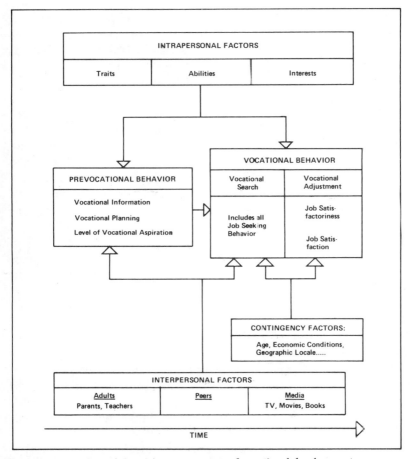

Figure 1. An outline of the major components of vocational development.

edge of the world of work, the amount of vocational planning he has engaged in, and the level of his vocational aspirations. External factors governing the client's behavior include both sources of information about jobs and work in general, obtained from parents, teachers, peers, etc. and several contingency factors, including age, current economic conditions, and geographic locale.

LIMITATIONS OF DEVELOPMENTAL RESEARCH

In order to investigate a global construct such as "vocational adjustment" or "family environment," the researcher must specify aspects of the construct that he feels are most important or that symbolize that area most accurately. The researcher must also be sure, as far as possible, that the aspect is defined clearly enough that it can be seen by any trained person through observation or direct measurement. Most survey research involves comparatively large numbers of subjects seen for relatively small amounts of time at widely separated periods. Therefore, the discrete item must be available from all subjects for study during a short time period. The final items which are to represent a general construct have passed through a selection process which may leave important information out of the research because it is too subjective, too transitory, too general, or not available on request. We all operate at a similar disadvantage of trying to build a total picture from limited information. The physician taking a pulse or the counselor conducting a screening interview is selecting specific identifiable aspects that are "symbolic" of more general functioning. The constraints on research are much greater.

For example, a significant relationship exists between the level of education of the mother and the time it took the subject to find employment. The higher the level of education, the longer time it took for the child to find a job. In attempting to understand the nature of this relationship, the following inferences could be made: (1) that better educated mothers set higher standards which the children have adopted (therefore the child is more selective and takes longer); (2) that the homes where there are better educated mothers tend to be more affluent (therefore, the family could support the subject financially for a longer period of time while he is seeking employment); and (3) that better educated mothers may be influential in the subject's receiving more post-high school training which, in turn, increases the selectivity of the student in obtaining initial employment.

Any or all of these inferences may be correct for the individual subject or the group taking longer in taking employment. There may be even more subtle interrelationships that are difficult to infer but may actually explain the relationship more fully. While results do show that certain aspects of the subject's environment have influenced a specific vocational behavior, the nature of the influence is sometimes more difficult to determine.

REVIEW OF VOCATIONAL
RESEARCH RELATING TO DEAF PERSONS

There has been a limited amount of research conducted relating to the vocational adjustment of the deaf. These studies have been confined to surveys of the vocational status of deaf workers. At the national level, Lunde and Bigman (1959) conducted the first large-scale survey of the occupational conditions of the deaf since the Martens (1937) survey. They obtained responses from over 10,000 deaf adults. Regional surveys were conducted by Boatner, Stuckless, and Moores (1964) in New England and Kronenberg and Blake (1966) in the Southwest, while Dunn (1957) conducted a survey of deaf workers residing in the state of Wisconsin. However, the majority of the surveys have been follow-up studies of former graduates of individual schools for the deaf: Central Institute (Hirsch, 1952), Kansas School (Mog, 1954), California School at Berkeley (Jacobs and Gunderson, 1957), Clarke School (Bruce, 1960), New York City Public School 47 (Justman and Moskowitz, 1963), and the Lexington School (Rosenstein and Lerman, 1963).

The major findings reported in the surveys may be grouped into six aspects of vocational achievement: occupational distribution, earnings, stability of employment, job satisfaction, training, and communication. On the average, over 60% of deaf adult males are employed in skilled or semiskilled occupations, while less than 10% find work in professional or managerial roles. Deaf women are reported to be employed in greater numbers in semiskilled or commercial occupations (55%), with fewer than 10% occupying professional or managerial positions. Over 20% of young adult males and women are reported to be working in unskilled roles.

Comparing salary levels between reported earnings of deaf adults and salary information available on the general population indicates that the level of earnings between hearing and deaf women is not significantly different. Deaf men earn less than hearing men. These findings may reflect underlying social trends. Women are usually trained for specific occupational roles which have little upward mobility (clerk, typist, secretary). Where the possibilities for greater mobility exist, as they do with males, deaf men tend to remain at the lower end of their occupational ladder.

In the past 20 years, following the general population trends, there has been a significant increase in job mobility among deaf workers. Earlier studies indicate high percentages (60–70%) of adult deaf workers were still employed in their first or second jobs. More recently, occupational surveys have indicated a significant increase in the number of job changes being reported. Six studies reported on the level of satisfaction deaf workers expressed regarding their jobs. One survey indicated that less than half of the respondents was satisfied. The remaining five studies indicated that, on the average, over 60% of deaf workers were well satisfied with their work. Salary and working conditions are indicated most often as reasons for the expressed satisfaction. There is a serious disparity between the vocational training received in schools for the deaf by deaf workers and their current occupational status. For the most part, the deaf adult workers described in the vocational studies have extremely limited opportunities for post-high school training other than on-the-job training. With limited opportunities for preparing deaf workers for a changing labor market, it is not surprising that an average of 65% are reported to be working in situations for which they had not received prior training.

Four studies investigated the methods of communication used at work. Professionals used speechreading and lipreading more than any other method, with the exception of teachers of the deaf who also used signing and fingerspelling. All other groups, craftsmen, clerical workers, and operatives, relied on writing. Signing was found useful by service workers and those in the unskilled labor categories.

The results of single survey research studies offer a surface picture taken at one point in time. They indicate current functioning and problems, but cannot define the developmental issues: how things get that way and where things might be headed. The studies that have been reviewed here offer a clear picture of deaf adult workers who are in the later stages of vocational development, the establishment or maintenance phases. Social changes, economic developments, changes in education, and changes in child-rearing practices that have occurred in the past 20 years may not yet be reflected in the pictures currently drawn of adult deaf workers. A more dynamic picture of vocational development is required to help determine the vocational functioning we can expect and to prepare for those services that will be required by the younger deaf members of the work force.

LEXINGTON VOCATIONAL STUDIES

For the past 13 years, the Research Department of the Lexington School for the Deaf has conducted four major studies related to vocational behaviors of deaf persons.

The initial study, "Vocational Status and Adjustment of Deaf Women" (Rosenstein and Lerman, 1963) (RD-601), the vocational adjustment of a group of former female pupils of the Lexington School for the Deaf, in attendance for varying periods during the years 1935–1957, was examined. A majority of these deaf women had made a successful adjustment on the job, and their vocational status aspirations and satisfaction were related to the specific school program they followed.

It was not possible to determine the relative contribution of the individuals' characteristics when they were children (that may have led to differential school placement by administrators) and/or the nature of the training program offered by a given school to the differences obtained. More detailed examination of prevocational operations and levels of vocational development of deaf students seemed warranted.

Therefore, a second project, "Vocational Development of Deaf Adolescents" (Lerman and Guilfoyle, 1970) (RD-1380), was concerned with delineation of the vocational development of deaf adolescents currently attending school. A model, based on the work of Super et al. (1957) and other relevant literature in the field, was developed. The model included an Index of Vocational Maturity, largely concerned with vocational information and vocational planning. It also postulated the development of relationships between vocational choice and vocational interest, abilities, intelligence, attitudes, and various measures of family background. The results indicate that the theoretical pattern of vocational development was sustained for the deaf. Subjects' vocational information and planning are related to their language and communication competence, the level of stimulation available in their home and, to a reduced degree, their intelligence and adolescent independence. Significant differences between deaf subjects and their hearing adolescent siblings were found on measures of prevocational behavior, although similar patterns with age were indicated.

The study suggests that existing programs for vocational training and orientation have little impact on deaf individuals. Deaf subjects, for example, from age 12 have incorporated subcultural stereotypes of deaf workers, with only limited amounts of information available to them about the vocational world.

The implications for vocational rehabilitation to be drawn from the results of this study, while clear enough, are such that attempts at rehabilitation may prove somewhat difficult to carry out. The results indicate that the vocational maturity of the deaf adolescent is primarily an outgrowth of his own language competence and of the cultural stimulation provided for him by his parents. Looked at more closely, what this means is that, since vocational maturity is essentially an index of an adolescent's fund of vocational information, the contributions of language competence and cultural stimulation can best be understood in terms of a *source of information* (a culturally stimulating environment must necessarily be "vocationally stimulating" as well) and the *ability to process information* (i.e., language competence). Both are essential since high language competence by itself cannot guarantee high vocational maturity unless the adolescent is provided with the necessary information. In a like manner, more availability of vocational information is no guarantee of vocational maturity unless the adolescent is capable of absorbing it.

From this point of view of vocational rehabilitation, this means that any attempt to improve the deaf adolescent's vocational maturity by supplying him with additional vocational information must give serious consideration to the problem of language competence. Insofar as strategy is concerned, that with the greatest potential involves an effort to upgrade and supplement existing language instruction programs in schools for the deaf since this will have the additional effect of creating opportunities for employment in areas previously closed to the deaf by virtue of their poor language skills. On the other hand, the interval between investment and payoff is likely to be several years, and it is likely that only the youngest deaf students will be the beneficiaries of such a strategy.

What is to be done with the older deaf students while this program is going on? Indeed, what is to be done with all deaf students if such a program proves impossible to implement? Obviously, a more realistic strategy is required either as a substitute for or supplement to the one above. One possible strategy entails the development of a standard vocational orientation program designed to supply vocational information and assistance through all available media. The goals of such a program (which could be offered to interested schools in a package form) would be: (1) to widen the deaf adolescent's vocational horizons by exposing him to as wide a variety of realistic vocational choices as is feasible (i.e., to break down the stereotype of "deaf job"); and (2) to provide relevant personal experiences for the adolescent expressing a specific vocational preference. For the past 3 years a program based on this concept, under the direction of the Rochester School for the Deaf, has been implemented in most of the special schools throughout New York State.

In a more recent project (RD-2453-S) (Lerman et al., 1969), the focus has shifted from the measurement of prevocational behavior to the measurement of vocationally relevant traits and interests of deaf adolescents. Ultimately, it was our intention to bring all of this work to bear upon the problem of the later work adjustment of the deaf adolescent.

There were three main objectives: (1) to determine the feasibility of using rating scale procedures for the measurement of vocationally relevant personality traits; (2) to determine the feasibility of using short, paper-and-pencil type tests to measure tolerances for several tasks and social demands imposed by the work situation; and (3) to construct an interest inventory which is more suitable for the deaf client and which provides the vocational counselor with more information about the client's interests.

The results on the development of a nonverbal interest inventory are incomplete and are still in the process of being validated. Nevertheless, from a tentative examination of the data, the results seem promising. Regarding the use of short paper-and-pencil tests for measuring various task and social tolerances presumed to be associated with job competence (routine, detail, frustration, novelty, ambiguity, distraction, and criticism), the results indicate that these tests are not valid measures of these types of behaviors. Rating procedures for measuring vocationally relevant personality traits may be used by the vocational counselor with a relatively small number of items (10–15) or can be obtained from teachers for reasonably reliable and valid estimates of the vocationally relevant traits of agreeableness, assertiveness, and intelligence. Such items may be administered individually to deaf clients to obtain self-ratings from them.

The most recent project (Guilfoyle et al., 1973) conducted by the staff of the Research Department of the Lexington School followed the group of students previously seen as teenagers into their young adult years. While many were hard to locate or still continuing their education, a sizable number of deaf subjects and their hearing siblings had entered the work force and were interviewed in the course of this study.

The results indicate that current vocational adjustment for a group of young adult deaf people is related to parallel behavior in their current situation as well as their prevocational behaviors. In analyzing four important aspects of vocational adjustment, including job satisfaction, job-seeking behavior, percentage of time employed, and percentage increases in salary, in terms of their relationship to other factors, it was found that more than 60% of the significantly related items were aspects of prevocational behavior or family background. These included expressed vocational interest, early vocational information, general intelligence and academic abilities, the number of deaf siblings in the home, high school graduation status, family cultural stimulation, and independent behaviors shown as adolescents.

EMERGING PROFILES OF DEAF WORKERS

By the age of 14, we can see emerging patterns among our students that have, in the past, crystallized into three general styles of later adult vocational adjustment. The student with marginal academic and language skills usually is directed into specific training on a semiskilled or unskilled level to work in filing, simple carpentry, sewing, or mechanical trades. He knows little of the general vocational picture and has either unrealistic or no plans for his future. Besides the immediate society of his deaf peers, he has no broad social experience or knowledge to help him adjust to the hearing community. The least competent of this group has trouble finding and maintaining himself in employment. The responsibility for his later vocational functioning rests with the family or with governmental or private agencies such as sheltered workshops. For this least competent segment, marriage and other intimate social relationships are difficult to develop and maintain. The students with marginal skills, but with good social and emotional functioning, find employment through their friends or through the schools. They are usually good workers who quickly find a job and, if they are reasonably comfortable, remain at the same place. But there is almost no advancement, and salary increase is limited. They marry, find other deaf people for friendship, and live in relative isolation from their community and coworkers. Deaf people in this group appear to be the most content and satisfied with their work. With limited skill and knowledge, their limited expectations are being met.

The student with good to excellent academic and language skills usually is directed into areas of further academic studies. Families of these deaf people can be characterized as being involved and interested, but not dominating. When this student completes his high school program he is directed toward post-high school training in college or technical institutes and schools. With average motivation and luck, he may try, after a longer job-seeking period, to find employment within his field of training or may resign himself to a position that is below his level of training but con- sidered good by standards of the general adult deaf community. With exceptional motivation and luck such a student may secure managerial and professional positions. For most members of this second group, good advancement and salary increases are possible. With good social, occupa- tional, and language skills they can interact with the hearing community and worker to gain acceptance which is required for advancement. While they spend more time in seeking and changing jobs, they do eventually establish themselves within well-defined vocational lines. This is a generally more aware group. They are sensitive to the potentials available in this society and to the restrictive prejudices of society. They are the most outspoken regarding their resentment about social barriers for the deaf. While they function on higher levels, their expectations are also quite high. They are not as well satisfied in their work as the group with marginal skills. They are vocationally well adjusted workers.

Disturbed family relationships and early emotional upsets are more common in the third group. At 14 years of age, members of this group have average to above average language and cognitive abilities, but have uneven or poor academic functioning. Some may complete high school and enter educational institutions for post-high school training, but frequently leave such training before completion. Others may be directed toward changing from an academically based program late in their high school education to a vocationally oriented one. Frequently the girls marry and leave school before graduation. For those who enter employment, personal, rather than economic, difficulties are related to job change. Many work at jobs below their abilities and may be considered occupational underachievers as they were educational underachievers. A number of this group are able to achieve emotional stability during their adult years and attempt to improve their occupational skills and redirect their careers. As a group, these deaf people are least satisfied and least vocationally adjusted.

Educators and counselors have had only limited experience with three subgroups: multiply handicapped, bilingual, and black deaf persons. Until recently, because of prejudice, lack of sufficient numbers, or subcultural attitudes, they have not obtained a reasonable share of consideration by service agencies or by the deaf community. These deaf groups, out of proportion to their numbers, would be found in the marginally functioning deaf worker group. There are indications in the last few years that greater consideration is being given to these subgroups. With greater effort and attention, the level of their functioning and development should improve.

SIGNIFICANT ISSUES

Vocational Training

The limited information that deaf adolescents hold and their limited opportunities to explore individual interests emphasize the need for increased vocational orientation activities. However, actual training in a particular skill or trade has been seriously questioned. A large number of deaf adults indicate that their earlier training was not useful in subsequent employment. For the deaf student with marginal abilities, where the general educational goal is that he be helped to maintain himself in a limited way as an adult, vocational training is important. It may be important for the more adequate functioning student under severe economic pressure. This student will need specific instruction on work-related language and social skills. While he may lack skills that will enable him to be flexible in his career, he will be able to enter and maintain himself at work. For most deaf students, specific vocational training may be started when they are too young. This training does not increase their knowledge about vocations in general or help them plan more thoughtfully about their futures. Without the students' sincere interest in what they will do when they go to work, such training seems wasted. Some skills courses have broad applicability—such as typing. Almost everyone can find a use for such a skill whether or not he chooses it for a career. The older adolescents are more anxious about their futures and have better understandings of reality factors that may affect their plans. It is at the point at which such planning is going on that meaningful vocational training can have its greatest impact. The greater the attention to the development of basic cognitive skills during adolescence, the more successful and flexible will be the worker. A number of students experience difficulty with programs of academic skills and they are, therefore, shifted to vocational training courses. For many, the difficulties are related to a lack of motivation or to the programing rather than an inability to further develop such cognitive skills. The same creativity that has been shown in the development of preschool programs must be channeled into program development for adolescents. Intensive vocational training in high school should be offered to those students who have a demonstrated need rather than as a ready alternate for students experiencing difficulties in academic work.

Vocational Rehabilitation Services

Social programing in the United States has attempted to create greater flexibility—and for specific groups which experience the greatest restrictive pressure (the poor, the culturally deprived, the mentally and physically handicapped) with limited success.

Deaf people have been influenced by federal, state, and local actions designed to extend the range of choice by improved education, educational opportunities, vocational training, and job placement. These activities do not affect deaf people equally. The more intelligent, skilled, and competent deaf person of today has far greater opportunities than he would have had 20 years ago. Part of vocational rehabilitation services with deaf people has been directed at this group, since these goals are readily attainable with a comparatively limited effort. Another group that has received attention has been extremely marginal deaf people whose difficulties are so evident that they must be responded to. They are sufficiently impaired for intellectual, social, economic, physical, and psychological reasons to bring them to the attention of local agencies. There are many more of these persons than appear for rehabilitation services since their family, neighborhood, or cultural groups are suspicious of government services. In most cases of this kind, "custodial" arrangements are developed.

Most deaf people we have interviewed during the past 13 years indicate very limited direct experience with governmental rehabilitation agencies. Few contacts in relation to job placement, vocational training, or counseling services are reported. Most of the recalled contacts with DVR counselors were to obtain financial aid to pursue post-high school education and training. The facilitating functions of referrals for evaluations, assistance in the establishment of training opportunities, working with schools and other service agencies on work-study and continuing education programs, or dealing with the business community to develop or expand opportunities for deaf workers are not known by members of the deaf adult community. While rehabilitation programs are being improved to meet the current need of this group, it is necessary to enlarge local contacts with the deaf community and its leaders to ensure their maximum effectiveness.

Socialization

The ability to develop good relationships with co-workers and supervisors and to communicate about the formal and informal aspects of work is extremely important in obtaining salary increases and promotions. The acquisition of a skill is necessary for obtaining a job, and salary (along with other benefits) is governed through contractual arrangements. The deaf worker with good social skills has greater opportunity to remain or to advance in his work. A deaf worker, having acquired the highest level of skill but lacking good social and communication ability, is virtually locked into a position and a salary. Many deaf teenagers appear to be socially immature, more dependent, lacking social knowledge, and exhibiting inappropriate social behaviors. This may be related to the home environment, their schooling, or the accepted norms of deaf peers. Reverse prejudice leads many adults to overprotect deaf youngsters, thereby reinforcing the social isolation and feelings of inadequacy that exist. Professionals offering services to deaf people can assist them in becoming less dependent and passive, more assertive, cooperative, socially knowledgeable, and socially skilled people. The acquisition of what appears to be "native abilities" is work. In the formative years, programing to ensure greater exposure to normally hearing individuals and groups at play, school, and work can be developed. Appropriate integrated settings can improve social competence and confidence. Since most deaf adults work with hearing co-workers and supervisors and since the social aspects of the work environment are important elements, they are at a vocational disadvantage if their social functioning is poor.

Language

Language is an essential feature of current adult functioning. The ability to read and understand written materials becomes increasingly critical as technological developments reduce the number of semiskilled occupations. In time, the less competent deaf person may be forced into the unskilled worker category, leaving only the more linguistically competent deaf group able to enter the technical, managerial, and professional occupations. Two types of linguistic competence can be delineated, one necessary for processing formal information and one necessary for social communication. For normally hearing people, competence in social communication using standard English is assumed. Recently, this assumption has been challenged because of large numbers of non-English-speaking people and large numbers of other people who speak dialects that are radically different from standard English. The emphasis in general education is to develop competence in reading and writing using spoken English as a base.

Since there are many people who do not benefit from current systems for teaching reading, emphasis is now being placed on programs that will teach reading skills and teach language systems at the same time. These approaches hold the promise of improving reading skills and knowledge of standard English for deaf people. Improvement in these areas is essential since the educational requirements for many jobs are increasing. Social communication is important on the job. Deaf workers have been able to work out systems with co-workers and supervisors to communicate on important matters. If the system is good, the flow of information will be easier and fuller. There will be greater job opportunities for the good communicator.

Early Evaluation

Considering vocational adjustment as one of the end points along a continuum of vocational development assists us in examining the influences that lead to any maladjustments. Our research indicates that prevocational behaviors are predictive of subsequent adjustment. Lack of vocational information and planning, poor development of interests and aptitudes, limited home stimulation, limited language development, poor social skills and attitudes, and the effects of long-term institutionalization interfere with successful vocational adjustment. Further longitudinal research with additional groups of deaf people is required to obtain a clearer picture of the causes of later vocational problems. Professionals making short-term observations can predict problems for students who are socially isolated, severely emotionally disturbed, severely limited intellectually and cognitively, or severely physically disabled. Less obvious behaviors of adolescents may indicate the necessity for intervention. While some intervention techniques have been described, more are needed. Improved methods for evaluation of prevocational behaviors are required and need to be implemented. If vocational rehabilitation personnel could take on the added role of vocational development advocates while the student was still in early adolescence, they might offer impetus for this program development.

REFERENCES

Boatner, E. B., E. R. Stuckless, and D. F. Moores. 1964. Occupational Status of the Young Adult Deaf of New England and the Need and Demand for a Regional Technical-Vocational Training Center. Final Report, Research Grant No. RD-1295-S-64, Vocational Rehabilitation Administration, Department of Health, Education and Welfare, American School for the Deaf, West Hartford, Conn.

Borow, H. (ed.). 1964. *Man in a World at Work.* The Riverside Press, Cambridge, Mass.

Bruce, W. 1960. Social problems of graduates of an oral residential school for the Deaf. Unpublished Master's thesis, University of Utah.

Dunn, J. G. 1957. Report of Special Project to Study Wisconsin's Rehabilitation Problems Associated with Deafness. Rehabilitation Division, State Board of Vocational and Adult Education, Madison, Wisc.

Guilfoyle, G. R., F. H. Schapiro, L. Katz-Hansen, A. Lerman. 1973. *The Evaluation of Vocational Development of Deaf Young Adults.* Final Report, Project No. RD-14-P-55065/2, Social and Rehabilitation Services, Department of Health, Education and Welfare. Lexington School for the Deaf, New York.

Hertzberg, F., B. Mausner, R. Peterson, and D. F. Capwell. 1957. Job Attitudes: Review of Research and Opinion. Psychological Service of Pittsburgh, Pittsburgh.

Hirsch, J. G. 1952. Post-graduate adjustment of deaf children. Unpublished Master's Thesis, Washington University.

Jacobs, L. M., and R. Gunderson. 1957. A follow-up study of the graduates of the California School for the Deaf at Berkeley between the years 1940 and 1950. Unpublished Master's thesis, University of California.

Justman, J., and S. Moskowitz. 1963. A Follow-up Study of Graduates of the School for the Deaf. Bureau of Educational Program Research and Statistics, Publication No. 215. Office of Research and Evaluation, Board of Education of the City of New York, New York.

Kronenberg, H. H., and F. D. Blake. 1966. Young Deaf Adults, An Occupational Survey. Arkansas Rehabilitation Service, Hot Springs, Ark.

Lerman, A., and G. R. Guilfoyle. 1970. Pre-vocational Behavior in Deaf Adolescents. Final Report, Research Grant No. RD-1380, Division of Research and Demonstration Grants, Social and Rehabilitation Service, Department of Health, Education and Welfare. Teachers College Press, New York.

Lerman, A., G. R. Guilfoyle, J. Greenstein, and L. Katz. 1969. *The Development of Measures of Vocational Interests and Relevant Aptitudes for the Deaf.* Final Report, Project No. RD-2453-S, Social and Rehabilitation Services, Department of Health, Education and Welfare. Lexington School for the Deaf, New York.

Lunde, A. S., and S. K. Bigman. 1959. Occupational Conditions among the Deaf. Gallaudet College, Washington, D. C.

Martens, E. H. 1937. The Deaf and the Hard of Hearing in the Occupational World. U. S. Office of Education Bulletin No. 13, 1936. U. S. Government Printing Office, Washington, D. C.

Mog, H. M. 1954. A questionnaire survey of former students of the Kansas School for the Deaf to determine the relationship between their vocational training and their present occupations. Unpublished Master's thesis, University of Kansas.

Roe, A. 1956. The Psychology of Occupations. John Wiley & Sons, Inc., New York.

Rosenstein, J., and A. Lerman. 1963. Vocational Status and Adjustment of Deaf Women. Research Grant No. RD-601, Office of Vocational Rehabilitation, Department of Health, Education and Welfare. Lexington School for the Deaf, New York.

Super, D. E., J. O. Crites, R. C. Hummel, H. P. Moser, P. L. Overstreet, and C. G. Warnath. 1957. Vocational Development: A Framework for Research. Teachers College, Bureau of Publications, Columbia University, New York.

Super, D. E., and P. Overstreet. 1960. The Vocational Maturity of Ninth Grade Boys: Career Pattern Study. Teachers College Press, Columbia University, New York.

⑥ | Academic Achievement

HELEN S. LANE

Batteries of achievement tests have been in use in the public schools of the United States since 1923. They have been standardized on school populations from all parts of the United States, from large and small urban areas and rural populations. Test items have been selected from textbooks used throughout the country and equivalent forms of the tests have been developed. Scores are usually expressed in terms of grade equivalents based on a 10-month school year and in terms of educational age.

The use of batteries of achievement tests enables us to compare the progress of deaf children with hearing children in public schools. The average scores for hearing children show uniform progress from year to year at a steady rate of growth. Scores for hearing-impaired children show a slower rate of progress, especially in tests requiring language skills.

Readiness for an achievement testing program can be determined by giving a first grade reading test. Batteries for achievement tests are usually published for grade levels as follows: primary (2–3); intermediate (4–6), and advanced (7–9).

The results of an annual achievement testing program can be used advantageously by school administrators, teachers, and counselors as a measure of annual progress. They aid in homogeneous grouping of children in classes, in decisions concerning job and class placement, as a guide in the provision for individualized instruction or in providing diagnostic teaching, and for conferences with parents and clients. Test scores serve also in comparison with national norms.

Most batteries of achievement tests are made up of tests of reading usually measured by paragraph meaning and word meaning; tests of arithmetic are usually divided into tests of computation and of problem solving, arithmetic concepts, or reasoning; tests of spelling which may be dictated for lower grades but involve multiple choice visual recognition at intermediate and advanced levels; tests of social studies and of science; and tests of language made up of sections on grammar, punctuation, capitalization, etc. There is some confusion in the interpretation of language scores to parents and to teachers of hearing children who have been told that language is the most difficult subject for the deaf because deaf children score higher on this test. The language test in a battery of achievement tests is based on grammatical errors of hearing children. Deaf children do not learn these errors and are well educated in formal grammar. For example, a deaf girl asked the examiner the meaning of "ain't" in a test sample because her teacher did not teach that word!

If classes of deaf children are placed in a regular elementary school, the administrator may question the slower progress of this group of children. Parents may blame the teacher or even their child for failure to progress in some subjects. There may be a plateau in tests requiring reading comprehension and reasoning at second grade level which is caused by the need for establishing a firm language foundation on which more concepts can be built and the vocabulary essential for such concepts be developed.

In rehabilitation counseling, the academic level of the client plays an important role for diagnosis and in placement for further education and job training. When counseling the deaf, a comparison with hearing norms serves as a guideline for expectations for success in placement. Knowledge of the reading level of a client will assist in the selection of additional tests.

ACHIEVEMENT TESTS OF THE DEAF (1921–1975)

The educational achievement of deaf children and adults has been measured and reported by many investigators, including reports of individual schools, surveys on a national basis, case studies of one individual, longitudinal studies, comparison of tests, and relation to other phases of development and methods of teaching. To cover all of the studies would require a volume and, therefore, only a few pertinent studies are reported here to show a trend of results over the years and some of the problems demonstrated by achievement test results.

The first report of tests to measure educational achievement of the deaf was in a monograph by Reamer (1921) who completed the survey under the direction of Dr. Rudolph Pintner. A battery of educational tests selected from various authors was administered to 2,172 deaf children ranging in age from 10–18 who were enrolled in 15 state schools and 11 day schools. Reamer concluded that there was an educational retardation of 5 years and a grade retardation of 3½ grades. In his text on intelligence testing, Pintner (1931) said the deaf child was not suited for academic instruction and should be given industrial training.

Hall (1929) reported that students entering Gallaudet College were not quite up to ninth grade as measured on the Stanford Achievement Test. Tests were given to entering students annually with a gradual increase to tenth grade in 1932, as Fusfeld (1933) noted at the meeting of the International Congress of Educators of the Deaf.

Schick (1935) was interested in a study of Forms V, W, X, Y, Z of the Stanford Achievement Test to see if they were equivalent forms and if certain subjects were consistently more difficult. She found, as a result of 237 tests administered to students at Central Institute for the Deaf, an educational quotient of 83.9, indicative of an educational retardation of approximately 2 years. Alternate forms of the test were not equivalent for the deaf and this could be attributed to several variables such as vocabulary, teaching techniques, motivation, and changes of students in groups tested annually. The difficulty of reading and reasoning required in certain subjects resulted in consistently lower scores on all test forms.

In 1966, McClure summarized results of the educational achievement reported in several studies that added to the discouraging picture of academic retardation. The studies he included were those of Hester (1963) who tabulated grade scores of 1,104 students, 16 years old or older from 55 residential schools and nine day schools. The range of grades for the graduates was from 3.1–12.8 with a median grade of 7.9; for the non-graduates, the range was 0.9–10.5 with a median grade of 4.7.

Boatner (1965) collected data for 1,164 students 16 years old or older from 67 residential schools, 15 day, and 17 denominational and private schools for the deaf. Those who received academic certificates from the residential schools had a grade average of 8.2 and those receiving vocational certificates had an average of 5.3. The day schools were combined with denominational and private schools and, for these, Boatner reported a grade of 7.3 for academic graduates and 5.0 for those who received vocational certificates.

The North Carolina School requested educational achievement scores for the top 10% of students graduating from 26 residential schools for the deaf. The grade average for this group of 728 was 7.7. This report included a statement of advancement of students of only two grades between the ages of 12 and 18.

As a final study in McClure's summary, he examined achievement scores of 334 students who left the Indiana School for the Deaf from 1954–1965. The average grade for the total group was 6.4, with a range of average grades from 4.6 for those receiving certificates to 8.3 for those receiving academic diplomas.

In March 1964, the Secretary of Health, Education, and Welfare appointed an Advisory Committee on the Education of the Deaf, with Dr. Homer Babbidge, Jr., President of the University of Connecticut, as Chairman. The report of this committee (1965) opened with the following summary statement: "The American people have no reason to be satisfied with their limited success in educating deaf children and preparing them for full participation in our society. . . . This unsatisfactory state of education of the deaf cannot be attributed to any lack of dedication of those who teach and work with the deaf. The basic explanation lies in our failure to launch an aggressive assault on some of the basic problems of language learning of the deaf through experience or well-planned and adequately supported research, and in our failure to develop more systematic and adequate programs for educating the deaf at all levels."

As a recommendation of this report, a National Advisory Committee on the Education of the Deaf was created under Public Law 89-258 in October of 1965 to report to the Secretary of Health, Education, and Welfare.

The Office of Demographic Studies of Gallaudet College received a grant from the Office of Education, United States Department of Health, Education, and Welfare for annual surveys of hearing-impaired children and youth. Data from the first survey were published in 1969 and included statistics of the results of the Stanford Achievement Test that was administered in the spring of 1969 to deaf children in 70 schools and 39 classes—a total of 11,544. There was no control of testing procedures beyond the printed instructions of the test, and the tests were machine scored. The grade level of the test was selected by chronological age as shown in Table 1. Results are reported for all tests in the battery according to chronologi-

Table 1. Stanford Achievement Test

Test level	Chronological age in years	Grade equivalents based on norms for hearing
Primary I	7–11	1–2
Primary II	11–14	2–3
Intermediate I	12–16	4–5
Intermediate II	13–17	5–6
Advanced	15–19	7–9

cal age and hearing level. Total reading scores ranged from 1.68 for the 7-year-olds tested on Primary I to 5.88 for 17-year-olds taking the Advanced test. In Arithmetic, grades ranged from 1.45 to 7.44. Reading is considered the most difficult test for the deaf, and arithmetic computation is the test that involves the least language.

In the survey given in the spring of 1971 by the Office of Demographic Studies, the test level most valid for each student was determined by scores on a reading pretest. The Stanford Achievement Test Form W was administered with Table 2 showing test level selected and scores.

It should be noted in Table 2 that, determined by the pretest, 70.6% of the deaf children in the United States were tested at Primary levels (grades 1–3), and they ranged in age from 6–20+ years.

Table 2. Stanford Achievement Test Form W test levels and scores

Test level	Range of grade norms for hearing	Deaf tested (%)	Median chronological age of deaf	Grade equivalents	
				Reading	Arithmetic
Primary I	1.5–2.5	35.6	11-2	1.88	1.77
Primary II	2.5–3.9	35.0	13-4	2.67	3.71
Intermediate I	4.0–5.5	16.9	14-9	3.86	5.12
Intermediate II	5.5–6.9	8.2	16-9	5.10	6.44
Advanced	7.0–9.9	4.3	17-6	7.33	8.35
All batteries	N = 17,000			3.02	4.09

Balow and Brill (1975) made a study of educational achievement test scores of 16 classes who graduated from the California School for the Deaf (Riverside). A full grade of progress on the total battery was recorded from the 1956–1959 group (grade 6.34) to the 1969–1971 group (grade 7.31). The highest battery score was 7.91 in 1966–1968.

In summary, there has been some slight improvement in educational achievement of the deaf, but the educational retardation is still one of the greatest barriers to academic and vocational success of the deaf.

PROBLEMS OF TEST SELECTION

Vocabulary of Instructions

The tester should check batteries of tests to be certain that the student will not fail because he does not understand what he is to do. If the test selected is too difficult, instructions may need to be rewritten or the vocabulary taught before testing.

Selection of Appropriate Grade Level for Valid Measure

Frequently the selection of the grade level is made by the classroom teacher or the supervising teacher.

A pretest of reading readiness may serve as a more reliable method of determining readiness for testing (e.g., Gates-MacGinitie Test) or a short reading test as was used in the National Survey.

Elliott and Healy (1970–1971) suggested that suitability of test difficulty may be determined by comparing observed test scores with scores expected by chance. Correction for guessing is not included in the scoring system for most batteries of tests. If a child's test score exceeds "the expected grade score," one may conclude that the test is valid. If the grade score is below or at "the expected grade score," the score is not readily interpretable, especially if all test items were not completed.

One of the modifications planned by the publishers of the revised Stanford Achievement Test for Hearing Impaired is adjusting of levels so that a student will receive reading tests at a level commensurate with his ability along with higher level tests in mathematics and spelling.

Dictated Test Items

At primary grade levels, many achievement tests are adding sections that must be dictated orally to meet the methods of instruction that are primarily oral and to be a better test for educationally disadvantaged children. To use these test items for the deaf, the standardization may be altered if they are given in sign language or in fingerspelling. If standard procedures are used, lipreading skills are tested in addition to the subject matter of the test. A spelling test given in fingerspelling cannot be considered a test of spelling ability! Test batteries must, therefore, be screened carefully in order to select one free of dictated items or to select one from which the dictated items can be omitted from the test when scoring without upsetting the value of the test.

In a pilot study in the spring of 1973, the dictated items of the Stanford Achievement Test were printed in a form for the hearing impaired. It was decided that the hearing impaired form did not present an advantage and because of the added cost it would not be used in the 1974 test revision. In the present Primary level of the Stanford Achievement Test, the section on word study skills and listening comprehension is questionable for use with the deaf.

Use of Partial Test

When testing time becomes a factor in deciding about the advisability of the use of an achievement test, certain parts of the battery may be selected. This occurs in rehabilitation counseling and in evaluation of children for admission to a school. Of course, the total battery is always preferable, but this may require 6 hours of testing time that must be appropriately spaced to avoid fatigue.

The reading tests and the arithmetic reasoning test give the best index of abilities necessary for academic or job placement, although these tests account for the maximum amount of educational retardation.

SUGGESTIONS FOR TEST ADMINISTRATION

Achievement tests can be given to a small group; in schools, the size of the group should not exceed 12–14 students. Assistants may help the psychometrist who gives the test. They are supplied with extra pencils and should move quietly around to be sure the child turns to the next page of the test when he has finished a page and does not start the next test until the instructions are given. The assistants must be cautioned not to hover over a child while he is taking the test.

Time limits for an achievement test are usually ample, but must be adhered to carefully. A flick of the light switch serves as a good signal for starting and stopping. In schools, tests should not be planned to terminate just in time for recess, lunch, or the close of classes. Children become tense if they are afraid they cannot finish in time for the above listed important events on their schedule!

The tester must be certain that the person to be tested understands the vocabulary of the instructions. For example, if, on the first page, he is told to write first name, middle initial, last name, is he confused by "middle initial"? Does he know the word "age" or is it better to say, "How old are you?" Be sure to write the date the test is given on the chalk board. Many of us get confused on calendar dates.

Does the testee understand the instructions at the beginning of each test? For example, "draw a circle around," "underscore," "fill in the space," "mark." These can be taught in the classroom. The use of an answer sheet for machine scoring may need additional explanation.

Samples should be copied from the test booklet or on the chalk board for each test in the battery, with a dramatic demonstration of the selection of the correct response, elimination of wrong answers, and filling in the correct space to record the answer. A child may be asked to demonstrate the second sample before testing begins.

The Stanford Achievement Series has now included a practice test at beginning levels.

Tests should be given preferably by the school psychologist, psychometrist, or the rehabilitation counselor. There is a tendency for classroom teachers to feel that the test is a measure of their teaching skills and not a measure of the child's knowledge, and they show undue concern while the child takes the test.

If test results are to be used as a measure of annual progress, the test must be given at the same time each school year.

If results will be used for diagnostic teaching or guidance, hand scoring is better than machine scoring. For example, if children consistently fail arithmetic problems involving more than one step by answers involving the first step only, the teacher can be sure they are not reading the whole problem.

An example of language confusion in arithmetic reasoning is in the interpretation of "more" which means addition to the deaf child. However, if a problem states that John has five dollars and Bill has three dollars and then asks how much *more* money does John have, his answer may be eight dollars. Subsequent teaching is needed to explain that subtraction is necessary to get the correct answer, and the teacher sees this need by studying the responses to the test.

Machine scoring is advised only when there is a large population to be tested, such as national surveys, and if only the subtest scores are important.

SUGGESTIONS TO REDUCE GAP BETWEEN INTELLIGENCE AND EDUCATIONAL ACHIEVEMENT OF THE DEAF

Most of the studies since the early 1930's indicate that the intelligence of the deaf is quantitatively normal, and performance test results show a normal distribution of intelligence quotients, but the educational level is from 2–5 years below normal expectancy. There have been many suggestions of ways to narrow this gap.

Early Identification and Early Education

The value of preschool education for deaf children was stressed as early as 1914 by Dr. Max Goldstein, when his first four pupils were of preschool age (3–4 years). Now, with early identification of deafness through the use of brain waves and computers, education may begin in the first months of a child's life. This is accomplished through programs of parent education either in the child's home or a simulated home situation. Results indicate that the early education programs result in earlier integration into classes for the hearing at normal grade levels.

In some instances, higher academic levels are reported for deaf children of deaf parents. Deaf parents usually do not have a course in teaching their deaf babies, although it is helpful for those who do. In the opinion of the author, the academic success of deaf children of deaf parents can be attributed to the early education of the child. They have experienced the educational procedures and communicate with their babies (orally or manually) from birth on. They always establish eye contact and they never stop communicating.

Maximal Use of Residual Hearing

Early identification of hearing impairment makes possible the early use of hearing aids. The use of amplification and the auditory training to perceive speech and environmental sound leads to improved listening skills as well as speech and language acquisition.

Reading for Recreation

Deaf children who read for fun are usually the ones who succeed in integrated programs. Scores on reading tests are the poorest in any battery of achievement tests of the deaf, and the lack of motivation to read can be explained by vocabulary problems and reading levels below the interest level. How much would we enjoy reading a novel in a foreign language if we had to hunt for the meaning of most of the words in a dictionary and then select from multiple meanings the one that fits?

In a study of reading scores of students at Central Institute for the Deaf, Lane and Baker (1974) reported a retardation of 2½ years and a gap of 33 points between IQ and educational quotient (EQ). The optimistic way to look at these data is that there was an improvement of 2.5 grades in a period of 4 years as contrasted with a gain of 8 months between the ages of 10–16 as reported by Wrightstone, Aranow, and Muskowitz (1963). The terminal reading grade for eighth grade graduates was 6.2 (not third grade), with the curve steadily rising and no evidence of a plateau. The scores used in this study did not include those deaf children who were integrated into hearing schools before they received five consecutive achievement tests.

Parental and sibling example plays an important role in motivation to read. With the increase in television viewing, there has been a decrease in recreational reading in many homes. Deaf children and their parents need guidance in the selection of reading materials, use of public libraries, and methods of stimulating reading interests dependent upon the age and interests of the child.

Development of Reasoning

Hall (1929) attributed some of the educational retardation of Gallaudet College students to lack of opportunity for problem solving. This is true today. Parents and teachers of hearing-impaired children think for them, anticipate and avoid errors, and prevent the child from learning through trial and error. The justification is that there is so little time to learn so much—and the deaf child grows up without the experience he needs to attack new problems without the fear of making mistakes.

Acquisition of Language

The major problems resulting in educational retardation of the hearing impaired are vocabulary, multiple meanings of words, verbalization of abstractions, and the complexity of the structure of our language. It is the teacher's task to develop language in deaf children who do not have the sensory channel that is considered essential for its acquisition. Language must serve a purpose, and schools and homes should create an atmosphere encouraging the use of language and reading.

RECOMMENDATIONS

Educational achievement tests should be given annually in schools for the deaf from second grade level until the student terminates his special education program. Results of these tests will give the administrator and teachers valuable information about progress in school subjects, will aid in homogeneous grouping, and will guide decisions concerning special tutoring.

Achievement test scores are sometimes prerequisites for admission to classes for the hearing and serve, along with other measures, as an aid in making decisions concerning readiness for integration. Grade norms help the teacher maintain a perspective about the progress of deaf children in special classes as compared to national grade levels for the hearing children of comparable chronological age.

Rehabilitation counselors need information about the academic skills of clients. Achievement test scores alert them to reading problems, vocabulary deficiencies, mathematical skills, etc. that will guide them in recommendations for vocational training, job placement, essential tutoring, or continuation of an academic program.

The Stanford Achievement Test is most frequently used in schools for the deaf. The American School Achievement Series has been used at Central Institute for the Deaf because there are no dictated items, the reading tests seem to require more reading for understanding with less opportunity for matching, and the vocabulary of instructions seems to be easier. The Metropolitan Achievement Series has norms for the deaf as well as for the hearing.

Whether achievement tests are used in a vocational counseling program or a school counseling program for guidance of the hearing impaired, the precaution should be observed that a child should never be promoted to failure and a deaf adult should never be placed where he is least likely to succeed because of academic limitations.

REFERENCES

Advisory Committee on the Education of the Deaf. 1964. Education of the Deaf. A Report to the Secretary of Health, Education, and Welfare. U. S. Department of Health, Education, and Welfare, Washington, D. C.

Balow, I., and R. Brill. 1975. An evaluation of reading and academic achievement levels of 16 graduating classes of the California School for the Deaf (Riverside). Volta Rev. 77:255–267.

Boatner, E. B. 1965. The Need of a Realistic Approach to the Education of the Deaf. Paper presented at a joint convention of the California Association of Parents of Deaf and Hard-of-Hearing Children, California Association of Teachers of the Deaf and Hard-of-Hearing and the California Association of the Deaf, Nov. 1965. (Cited in McClure, 1966.)

Elliott, L., and W. Healy. 1970–1971. Selection of achievement test level for hearing impaired children. In Language, Speech and Hearing Services in Schools. American Speech and Hearing Association. No. 5, pp. 33–42.

Fusfeld, I. 1933. What Standard Tests Have Shown at Gallaudet College. pp. 197–206. Proceedings of the International Congress on the Education of the Deaf, Trenton, N.J.

Goldstein, M. 1933. Problems of the Deaf. The Laryngoscope Press, St. Louis, Mo.

Hall, P. 1929. Results of recent tests at Gallaudet College. Amer. Ann. Deaf 74:389–395.

Hester, M. 1966. Manual Communication. Proceedings of the International Congress on Education of the Deaf, 1963, pp. 211–221. Gallaudet College, Washington, D.C. (Cited in McClure, 1966.)

Lane, H., and D. Baker. 1974. Reading achievement of the deaf: Another look. Volta Rev. 76:279–291.

McClure, W. 1966. Current problems and trends in the education of the deaf. Deaf Amer. 18:8–14.

Office of Demographic Studies. 1969. Academic Achievement Test Performance of Hearing Impaired Children, United States. Series D, No. 1. Gallaudet College, Washington, D. C.

Office of Demographic Studies. 1971. Academic Achievement Test Performance of Hearing Impaired Children, United States. Series D, No. 9. Gallaudet College, Washington, D. C.

Pintner, R. 1931. Intelligence Testing, Chapter 15. Holt Co., New York.

Reamer, J. C. 1921. Mental and educational measurements of the deaf. Psychol. Rev. Monogr. 29 (3).

Schick, H. 1935. A five year testing program to measure the educational achievement of the deaf. Oralism and Auralism, June, pp. 5–16.

Wrightstone, J. W., M. S. Aranow, and S. Muskowitz. 1963. Developing reading norms for deaf children. Amer. Ann. Deaf 108:311–316.

TESTS

American School Achievement Test. The Bobbs-Merrill Co., Indianapolis.
Metropolitan Achievement Test. World Book Company, New York.
Stanford Achievement Test. Harcourt, Brace, and World, Inc., New York.

7 | Psychiatry and Problems of Deafness

KENNETH Z. ALTSHULER

Psychiatrists were little interested in the problems of deafness before the 1950's. There were a few reports on traumatic deafness occurring in war, but other articles were rare. And those that were available were usually theoretical webs spun from an armchair, and indicative of little contact with real deaf persons. In some papers, one could not distinguish whether the topic was early total deafness or the deafness or partial hearing impairment of a later stage of life. Such differences, of course, are crucial to an understanding of consequences attributable to the handicap, for the handicap, like a drought, affects seedlings differently than full grown oaks and has different effects if it is partial or total.

This chapter will focus on early and profound deafness only. Hearing loss in adults or the elderly, whether it is chronic or acute, or partial or profound, influences a personality that is already formed; the sequelae depend for the most part on how well the individual was integrated before the accident, illness, or other cause of loss. In early total deafness, the absence of audition is present from near the beginning of life and affects all systems of adaptation, both as they develop and in the end result achieved.

The perspective of psychiatry holds that the child is father to the man. One enters life with a genetic endowment that frames the limits. One person could be a genius, another cannot. Some can grow to 6 feet, 2 inches, others have no chance. Men and women will be different in ways that both sexes find satisfying and aggravating, simply because of the genes and chromosomes they carry. Within this frame, life's experiences—in the family, physical, and even nutritional environment—determine where in the range of his potential a person will ultimately fit.

Early experiences, because they are first and because the developing child is immature and malleable, are the largest forces in this development. And when a fork in the road is taken, the further path and end result are naturally, and perhaps irrevocably, altered. Children with rickets (vitamin D deficiency), for example, may never develop bones that are fully straight even if the vitamin balance is later restored, and animals reared in darkness for the first few months of life will fail to integrate vision into their adult responses in dangerous situations. Clearly, interaction between heredity and environment begins early—even in intrauterine life—with the influence of one so intertwined with the other as to be, for practical purposes, inseparable later in life.

The wisdom of evolution has also arranged for human beings to mature and develop in a sequential fashion. The program has it that a newborn cannot control his senses nor all his musculature. As the biological sequences come into play, he will smile, then sit, then teethe, and later crawl, then walk, and speak. His environment is neatly suited to support and respond to this progress, yet must cope with it as well. The newborn's helplessness inspires tender care. His smile rewards a mother who is tiring, and events like sitting and the first words and steps evoke a satisfaction that is reciprocal and which forms the matrix for sound psychological development. Without this matrix of care (if babies are given only the physical necessities of food and a perfunctory diaper change, but are not handled lovingly), infants fail to thrive and may even die. As mobility and self-awareness come into play, the environment must encourage while it trains. Language emerges at this juncture, a fortuitous tool to import meaning to restrictions and generate a proper balance of closeness and separation.

All of this presumes that the child and parent are each equipped for their anticipated roles. Hence, the concepts of average expectable environment and average expectable equipment: the one suggests that a family is the place best suited for a child and the other that an intact child is most likely to reap the best from an expectant family.

A child that deviates from the expected in some particular will tend to unbalance the natural program. Imagine, for example, the parental response to a child that does not smile. While the smiling response of the deaf child appears on schedule, his babbling falls off at about 6 months; and sometime thereafter parents begin to feel an uncomfortable sense that something is amiss. The diagnosis of deafness is usually confirmed by the time the child is a year old (although a fourth of the time, the first doctor consulted does not properly evaluate the situation). Parents' reactions and how they impinge upon the child's development are legitimate interests of psychiatry. Since such reactions persist and have played a molding role in the adult deaf person who presents himself for help, they should be understood by vocational counselors as well. Of equal importance to psychiatrists and counselors are how the absence of sound—and truncation of the functions it serves—may limit or alter the usual developmental path.

Psychiatric inquiry into a number of these questions began some 20 years ago, when the Federal Vocational Rehabilitation Administration approached a research group from Columbia University with questions about how to deal with the emotional problems that seemed to limit successful rehabilitation in many of their deaf clients. Starting from scratch, the research team did a census of the deaf throughout the state of New York, conducted depth interviews of a sample of 300 normal deaf persons, studied such special groups as deaf offenders, achievers, and hospitalized psychiatric patients, and, most importantly, opened the country's first mental health out-patient clinic for deaf patients. From these beginnings, a gradual widening of interest developed, nationwide and internationally, so that there are now special psychiatric facilities for the deaf, not only in New York, but also in Washington, D. C., California, Illinois, and Wisconsin, and in Great Britain, Norway, Sweden, and Yugoslavia. While the bulk of the work has been with deaf adults, there is a sufficient body of experience to allow inferences about what distinguishes the deaf child's path of development on his way to adulthood.

NORMAL DEVELOPMENT AND CHARACTER

We have posited that the child is father to the man. Before turning specifically to deafness, let us review briefly the normal milestones passed in this trajectory. In the first year of life, the child is helpless, absolutely dependent for sustenance on the world about him and unable yet to distinguish where it ends and he begins. His first task, then, is that of attachment, to bind himself to those who nurture. He is equipped only with the charm of his helplessness and a few reflexes: rooting (searching for the breast with his mouth), grasping, and the startle reflex. Gradually he develops additional equipment: he lifts his head, he smiles, he coos, he giggles, and he sits. As rudimentary as they are, these tools suffice; the parents respond, and each step is welcomed as the miracle of growth which, in truth, it is.

From the psychological view, we imagine that the child's sense of himself at this time is one of omnipotence. Discomforted, he cries and magically relief appears. To get through this period in good health, the magic must work with some consistency. If the cries evoke no response or an extremely uncertain one, the basic relationship with the world is disturbed, and basic trust—a sense of safety in being and being with others—does not take root firmly.

In the second half of the first year of life, differentiation of self and object (the self as opposed to the world around and the people in it) begins. The stranger anxiety of about 7 months—a fear of strangers and tearful clutching of the mother in their presence—reflects an awareness that there are others, not all of whom are alike. The awareness marks the commencement of separation—individuation, the establishment of a sense of separate identity which is the primary task of the next 2–3 years.

Through maturation, the child's armament for this job has been considerably augmented by 1½ years: he knows clearly that there are others than himself, and he is capable of internal representations of them symbolically so that he knows they exist even when out of sight (while before this time, it was as if objects out of the immediate perceptual field were never there and gone forever). With this ability, he is even capable of simple ideas of space, time, and causality.

So, he sees himself as separate. And he has also progressed through crawling to walking, and has, therefore, the means to put distance between himself and others. Neither separation nor mobility is entirely a blessing. Being separate, he also realizes he is small. He strays not too far from mother in increasing circles, but becomes frightened or angry if she leaves or is beyond the reach of an immediate recall. Separate, he is only still omnipotent and safe if it is he who controls mother and not the other way around. He tests his new-found "me-ness" and is oppositional or commanding. The "terrible 2's" (and 3's) commence, and the battle of who is boss is on. With his newly developed mobility, he explores his world, at the same time getting into everything, leaving a mess behind him, and being generally troublesome to all.

The 2's and 3's are also the time of toilet training, and much of the parent-child relationship can be typified or symbolized by issues around the battle of the potty. For the parent, the goal overall is to help the child to confident autonomy and self-control. She wants to socialize the tyrant, not through counter-terror, whereby fear alone controls the impulses, but in a manner that encourages the harmonious and comfortable internalization of her standards of control. She wants the child to love her, to want to please her, and to yield his prerogatives over feces, urine, and general disruptiveness for the reward of her smile and a sense of mutual accomplishment. Successfully traversed, the child leaves this stage with a sense of self and autonomy. In the face of too much terror, lack of understanding on either side, or deficiencies in feelings of a safe and close relationship, the child is left with doubt and shame, fearful compliance or automatic defiance, and a lack of individuation that makes him prone to indiscriminately continue the power struggles of this age with later parent surrogates.

From 4–6, it is the family romance that flourishes. The child has a full sense of himself, wants to show off his accomplishments and be a big man. Childhood sexual feelings emerge; he loves his mother (if a girl, her father) and wants her for himself—to the exclusion of siblings and the other parent. But this cannot be, and the anxiety engendered leads to fears of bodily integrity—evinced by over-attention to bandaids, bumps, and scratches—which are ultimately resolved by an identification with the parent of the same sex and a decision (not conscious) to look elsewhere for a love of his own. This is the well known stage of the oedipus complex, and a successful traversal yields a sense of initiative and pride, while failure leads to sexual inhibition and excess anxiety and guilt.

At this point, the child is packed off to school, and his horizons are enlarged to vistas beyond his immediate family. These new experiences consolidate the past successes and failures. They provide a great deal of interaction with peers, a chance to test oneself against others, to join and further identify with same-sexed pals, and the opportunity for disciplined work and augmentation of the skills of knowledge. From 6–12 is called the latency period because sexual interests seem to recede in favor of same-sex socialization, study, and learning. "No fraternization" is a cardinal rule that heightens same-sex identification, and other-sexual interest is greeted with jeers and teasing. Success in this stage gives the child a sense of self and a place in the world, and the skills of industry; failure breeds a sense of inferiority.

This is as far as we shall go in reviewing early development. Adolescence and adulthood, of course, come next, but most authorities agree that the cardinal aspects of character are laid down well before. Naturally, each phase colors and influences the ones succeeding: the child neglected for the first year enters the next stage less likely to trust, to love, and to yield without panic than one whose basic trust was encouraged. Similarly, excessive battles in the second and third years will color a child's perception of oedipal-sexual feelings with greater phantasies of violence and destruction than would be anticipated for one who learned impulse control less traumatically.

A few additional points are worthy of emphasis. On the one hand, no one comes through childhood unscarred, unbent, and without some idiosyncratic molding experiences. On the other, the child is a resilient little creature who can bounce back well if stresses are not too severe and persistent. Moreover, for each phase of development, the acceptable range of behaviors for both child and parent is broad; given half a chance, the forces of maturation and development will yield what might be called a normal adult neurotic—like most of us.

To summarize, we have noted that it is the quality of the child's attachment to the mother, then the course of separation-individuation coupled with the development of impulse control which are the first cornerstones in personality development. The course of these phases influences traversal of the oedipal and latency periods and what follows thereafter as well. The precise and inevitable effects of early total deafness on this development (and there must be some) are, quite simply, unknown. The basic situation is obviously at least as complicated as for the hearing, where qualities of children and parents vary along with variations in rates of growth and maturation. For the deaf, there are additional factors, such as when the handicap is discovered, how long it takes parents to get accurate guidance about what is required of them to minimize its implications, and the extent and quality of their own emotional reactions.

From experience with deaf adults and from what is known of normal development, some likely inferences can be made. Sound is an important part of the child's bond with his mother. He has, after all, only touch, vision, sound, and a primitive grasping (a part of touch) to make this bond at first. A mother's voice nearby will quiet an infant at only a few weeks of age, and cooing and talking, along with looking and touching, are important parts of the earliest nursing situation. While sound binds, it is also important in the later separation phase, for it uniquely maintains contact out of sight and at a distance. Sound further serves an important function in generating and modulating emotions. All of us throughout our lifetimes respond to music and rely on tonal qualities of speech to convey nuances and to arouse or dispel feelings. In situations of tenderness or anger, for example, the messages of tone are often more important than the messages of content. For suasion or persuasion, protestations of innocence or menace, tone is often the effector agent.

Sound is also the most abstract of our senses. Touch is totally concrete; to be informed by touch one must be in contact with the object, and only a small part of it can be apprehended at any given time. Vision offers distance and can scan the world in serial fashion, but each visual fix in the series is static and bound to the concrete picture. Sound, on the other hand, is omnidirectional. Through it, we scan the world continuously, covering simultaneously 360° around us. At the same time we separate the important from the unimportant, so as to react to one and ignore the other. As any city dweller besieged with nightly noise can tell, through sound we do this even while we sleep!

More commonly emphasized is the role of sound in the development of language. At about 1½, language begins to be acquired by anyone exposed to it. Several investigations have shown that language is not a requisite for thinking to develop. But sound generally—and by means of language particularly—is a major vehicle for conveying information which thinking can chew over, digest, and grow upon.

The person with early total deafness does without all of these attributes of sound (except for deaf individuals of deaf parents, for whom at least language (manual) is available and on time in the developmental schedule).

At least equally important in the development of the child is the reaction of his parents. About 90% of the deaf come from hearing mothers and fathers who are thoroughly surprised by the handicap. Carrying or siring a child is an emotionally laden experience—witness the fact that whatever the little ruffian really looks like, he is beautiful to his parents. He is their creation, a part and extension of themselves, and generally felt as destined to be and represent all the best they could have been. (Even in the disadvantaged and in the cases of child abuse, there is often an element of disappointed rage based on such expectations, e.g., the child is not the perfect plaything, the doll expected, but a demanding and, therefore, frustrating creature.) Readiness to love, which is partly a consequence of such feelings, enables the parents' part of the bond to build. Each response, each new milestone rewards and reassures their hopes, eliciting comfort, pleasure, and further pleasurable anticipation.

Unless there is reason for early suspicion (maternal rubella, for example), the first 6 months generally unfold in line with what the parents had in mind. Then, as the deaf child's babbling drops off or something fails to appear on the social schedule of 6–12 months, parents become uneasy. After a period of increasing anxiety and the discomfort of something vaguely perceived as strange, the diagnosis is made.

Depression is added to the anxiety; the child is not whole somehow. What is he, what is wrong with us, and what will he be, are the questions wrestled with. Ignorance (of causes and the consequences of deafness) heightens the pain and uncertainty, unleashing fantasies of damage and dementia that reach surrealistic heights through the force of disappointment. Handling that formerly was natural becomes strained.

If parents are lucky enough to find good counsel, they may obtain some relief. They can be helped to realize that deafness is, after all, only deafness; that their child is not dumb, in the sense of stupid, but that he just does not hear; that this will limit his experience, but that he is educable and otherwise healthy; that he will develop normally, given a chance; and that if they will learn manual language and substitute visual for verbal language, he will even have language skill and comprehension on a normal schedule; and that perhaps, if they encourage babbling and an interest in sound, and use amplification early and wisely, he may even be able ultimately to convert his natural interest in language and communication into useful verbalization.

Such counsel can effectively restore the parents' sense of comfort with the child and do much to preserve the nutrient matrix in which healthy development can flourish. Unfortunately, it has been rarely available in the past, and a confusion of guidance was the rule. Parents seek to relieve their unhappiness by consulting a variety of experts. Their effort is to deny the handicap and the bizarre consequences they guiltily imagine and ascribe to it. "If it is not seen, it isn't there" is an unconscious equation. The idea of manual language in full visibility is not easily accepted, therefore, unless they are educated to the readiness for language acquisition at about 1 year to 1½, and to the fact that manual communication can help, not hinder, the child's development, and that its use will enrich his life and be a supplement to, not a demotivation from, an interest in speech.

Parents of most patients and clients seen by psychiatrists and counselors in the past, and probably for the next 20 years, have not been so guided. Left to their own devices, and conflicted, they refract advice to encourage speech through the prism of their wish to deny the handicap. The result is such strange behavior as adults contorted out of shape to keep their lips at the eye level of a toddler, or stiffly shaping slow words with less hand movement clues than they would use with their other hearing children.

There are no villains in this scenario. For the most part, parents love and mean well for their youngsters. But there are conflict, guilt, denial, and ambivalence. And there is inadequate and piecemeal advice. Together they yield confusion and uncertainty in dealing with the deaf child. The spontaneity, the instinctive rightness and harmony of action-reaction between parent and child, is altered, and each phase of the developmental sequence outlined earlier is affected.

How to feel close to a child that is strange is a problem. How to encourage discipline and self-control based on loving communication, rather than fear, is a problem when communication is drastically limited. Logistical problems are innumerable: can he play in the front of the house where cars pass (unheard); can the family go to a movie together, which he will not hear; what to do when he can turn off an unpleasant admonition simply by looking away.

The deaf psychiatric patient or vocational client has often come through this overall obstacle course with the least success. A number of features are typical. He is usually language-poor in English. He is concrete in signs and naïve in general information, having been blocked from the vast range of auditory experience and being limited in both general and reading experience. As part of being naïve, and because education requires so much effort to get information into him that independent thought and conceptual exercises are often laid aside, he is frequently self-centered and dependently expectant that much will be done for and little required of him. His internal controls are often uncertain, a result of early confusion in relationships and either inconsistent, too severe, or faultily apprehended disciplinary experiences, so that under pressure he will behave impulsively or yield to temper. His sense of others, of his impact on them, and their legitimate expectations of him are often faulty.

In terms of our earlier discussion, it can be seen that the problems may very well not interfere with basic trust, the task of the first year. It appears, retrospectively, that most difficulties occur in the period of separation-individuation and autonomy. Interestingly enough, we have seen little of an excess of shame in our deaf patients. It is rather as if the internalization of impulse control was incomplete and there is a reliance (unconscious) on the continued ability of anger to coerce care or yielding from others. Perhaps the deafness, making unclear the early recognition of social disapproval, shame's precursor, limits its development.

All these statements, of course, are generalizations. As such, none is always correct, and none should be applied stereotypically or indiscriminately. The portrait is a composite, drawn from frequently recurring elements. Some clients or patients will show all of the features sketched, some will show none. As a shorthand, and for purposes of recall, the composite can alert the counselor to those elements of character which he is likely to encounter in his work with the deaf.

PSYCHIATRIC DISORDERS AND DEAFNESS

None of the characteristics noted above are unique to deafness. Many are found also in disadvantaged populations where, interestingly enough, poor language skills are the rule despite unimpaired hearing. Among the culturally disadvantaged, impulsivity, immaturity, and retarded language development derive from a poverty of parental concern and the absence of generally enriching experience. What is implied is that early profound deafness, without preventative and remedial measures, may interfere with normal parent-child relationships and life experience in general with a comparable result.

In cases of minimal brain dysfunction, the picture is also similar, but exaggerated. Affected youngsters are children with subclinical brain damage (i.e., minimal enough to be uncertain of detection on ordinary neurological examination) who are characterized by hyperactivity, poor impulse control and frustration tolerance, and limited attention span. As adults, they may continue to be impulsive or explosive and are generally brittle and self-centered.

Minimal brain damage often accompanies early total deafness since both may be caused by maternal rubella, encephalitis, or other etiological factors. And some deaf children are raised in disadvantaged homes and families. To the extent that either of these factors is present, the characteristics outlined as most common and typical of the deaf person in need of help are magnified.

Deafness is, of course, a perceptual handicap. It therefore alters life's experience for the deaf individual. But it does not necessarily protect him from life's conflicts nor limit whatever other genetic potentials he may carry. He is, therefore, with certain differences in form, as prone as anyone else to the standard variety of psychiatric ills.

Let us briefly review the psychiatric menu in a simple and diagrammatic fashion. A *neurosis* is a maladaptive way of coping with conflict, generally accompanied by or resulting in palpable internal distress. The model of neurosis is one of conflict. Unacceptable wishes or impulses, deriving from early life, are held out of awareness by repression. When stimulated by a new situation (touching on such prohibited areas as sex, aggression, or dependency, for example), the wishes threaten to burst into consciousness or overflow into action. Anxiety is generated in the face of this situation. If the anxiety is not bound by some new defense against it, *acute anxiety reactions* or a *chronic anxiety state* may appear. The former is an attack of panic, lasting from a few minutes to an hour, accompanied by tremulousness, rapid heartbeat, sweating, and an acute sense of dread or fear of death. The latter is a more chronic state of anxious expectation and inner tension, of lesser severity but with comparable fears that something bad is about to happen.

Such states are not easily borne, and the individual unconsciously seeks to bind the anxiety and avoid it by other defensive maneuvers. If it can be attributed to open spaces or closed (e.g., elevators, subways, or busses), or animals or other objects, then these situations or objects can be avoided; and by such constriction of lifespace, the anxiety is avoided too. This is the *phobic reaction.*

The anxiety can also be bound by symbolic displacement and *conversion reaction.* If the anxiety is caused by aggressive wishes to strike, for example, the right arm might become paralyzed, on a psychological rather than neurological basis. In such a case, the muscles that are "paralyzed" are not distributed in accord with any actual pattern of nerve innervation, but according to the function that their use may symbolize. The individual affected is often indifferent to his paralysis, presumably because it has relieved, rather than induced, some inner tension.

Another means of warding off the anxiety is by *obsessive-compulsive reactions,* in which obsessional or compulsive defenses are evoked, such as hand-washing rituals, counting, or turning off lights or faucets. Such rituals symbolize and act as a form of control. Often the anxiety threatens to break through nonetheless, and the rituals must be repeated or extended over and over, or there are obsessive recurrent thoughts or doubts that some aspect has been omitted or is insufficient to prevent impending catastrophe.

Riddance through action is also a means of dealing with anxiety. In these cases there are explosive reactions or impulsive acts designed to act against or get away from whatever is felt to be the cause of the unpleasant feelings.

Since the anlagen for obsessional reactions is laid down during the early training experiences and requires a solid set of internalized controls, and since these are the areas we have noted as generally (again with exceptions) weakest among deaf patients, such reactions are less common among the deaf than the hearing. As a corollary, impulsive behavior is more common.

The same can be said for the whole range of *character disorders.* Character disorders are deeply ingrained maladaptive patterns of behavior. The characterological qualities serve as an armor against childhood and later adult anxiety. Unlike the neurotic reactions, which are felt as foreign to the person, the character defenses work fairly well for the individual. They generally cause him little direct discomfort, but they may alienate or be experienced as unpleasant or hurtful by others, and indirectly can make for unhappiness in the affected individual. The *narcissistic character,* for example, relates to others only insofar as they feed his sense of being important and so is lonely or searching always for a new source of such stimulation. The *obsessional character* is rather brittle, meticulous to the extreme, and equally demanding of others. The *paranoid character* is suspicious of all. The *passive-dependent* and *passive-aggressive* characters may cling to or coerce care from those around them and be aggressive directly or through passive resistance when disappointed. Here again, among deaf patients, the obsessional character is rare (although most common among the hearing), the paranoid character—often related to the obsessional—is infrequent, while the more impulsive and passive-dependent and aggressive presentations are more common.

A common type of difficulty, in both deaf and hearing individuals, is the *situational maladjustment*. Here an otherwise sound individual is temporarily overwhelmed by the burden of circumstance. Among deaf clients such reactions often occur in relation to financial burdens or family or job problems. In younger deaf subjects, e.g., adolescents, they often eventuate from inordinate family pressures to achieve beyond the intellectual capacity or social opportunity afforded to the particular individual; in such circumstances, these reactions generally reflect a family problem in which parents are unconsciously denying the handicap and its limitations. The deaf youngster, being relatively silent, becomes the stage and unwitting victim through which the conflict is played.

The treatment in situational reactions must obviously be directed to the amelioration of the precipitating pressures, for which guidance, supportive counsel or therapy, and time are required. In cases of family reactions, treatment must often involve the whole family; resistance is inevitable and frequently makes the going slow. Psychiatric help may be necessary, and this is also the case where a neurosis or severe character disorder is involved. The counselor, however, should be able to roughly recognize the type of problem and work jointly with, or under the supervision of, a qualified psychiatrist. Minor tranquilizers and supportive, dynamically oriented psychotherapy are the tools which, buttressed by appropriate vocational counseling and placement, can lead to improved overall adjustment and functioning. Many deaf individuals in the neurotic range are amenable to some insightful psychotherapeutic work as well; to learn to appreciate the effects of their behavior on others, for example, to develop greater self-control, or to modify excessive expectations or demands of people they rely on. Modified forms of psychoanalysis have been used with a few patients, but their prerequisites in terms of frustration-tolerance, conceptual and communicative skills, and time make them seldom the treatment of choice for patients with early total deafness.

Life conflicts may also be integrated in a psychotic fashion. Most authorities now agree that a genetic predisposition is required for this to occur, at least insofar as the most common psychoses, *schizophrenia* and *manic depressive disease*, are concerned. The "split personality" of schizophrenia refers to a disintegration of function in the various aspects of personality (and not the multiple, complete personalities of popular fiction). Thus, the thoughts are disordered or loose in their connections and often make no surface sense. Or the affect, the emotional expression, is blunted, flat, hard to emphathize with, or out of phase with the ideas it accompanies.

Manic-depressive disease is typified by recurrent severe bouts of depression, sometimes in cycles in which mania occurs as well. In psychotic depression, the person looks sad and communicates slowly with a depressive mien. His movements and responses are retarded. There is weight loss, early morning wakening, and lack of interest in food, sex, or activity. Delusions of guilt over past and minor sins may be present or bodily delusions which express the depressive concern, e.g., a sense of "nothing inside" or of rotting away or being dead. Marked anxiety and agitation may also be a feature. The manic phase is characterized by inordinate energy, nonstop movement, flights of ideas and pressured speech (or other communication), with marked irritability in the face of efforts to interrupt the action or bring the person down to earth.

Schizophrenia occurs about equally in both sexes with an onset anywhere from 15–45 years of age. Manic-depressive psychosis is more common in women than in men. For the depressive type the peak age of onset is about 40, while in the mixed type (with bouts of mania as a part of the picture) the mean age of onset is in the early 30s. Both illnesses are often characterized by relapses and remissions. While in schizophrenia each attack may leave some residual impairment that interferes with functioning, in manic-depressive disease the individual is usually clear and able to return to functioning as before between bouts of illness.

Involutional psychosis occurs later in life, after age 45, and is thought to be associated with adaptive problems relating to the climacterium. It is more common in women than men and occurs in either a depressed or paranoid form. The depressive presentation may be of a slowed down type or one of agitation, with delusions of guilt and expiation. The paranoid form usually carries with it delusions of the type implied by the name.

Still later in life there are the *organic brain syndromes* of cerebral arteriosclerosis and senility, in which there are clouding of consciousness, disorientation, and general loss of intellectual functions, such as memory and judgment.

All these illnesses may occur in persons with early total deafness. The deaf, however, are generally relatively silent and their clinical presentations are often expressed in action rather than words and verbalized thoughts. In the majority of cases found in psychiatric hospitals, the bouts of illness leading to hospitalization were typified by impulsive, aggressive, or bizarre behavior, regardless of the diagnosis ultimately defined. The lack of words, the expression in action, the impulsive appearance which is widespread even in the less ill, and the expressivity inherent in manual language, all complicate the making of a diagnosis. Thus, except in the most flagrant cases, accurate diagnosis usually requires time and patience.

One striking finding has been the relative infrequency of slowed down forms of psychotic depression among the deaf. This does not mean that deaf persons do not become sad or depressed or even that psychotic levels of depressive reactions are infrequent. But the clinical presentation is altered. In the hearing, the presence of psychomotor retardation and guilty self-recrimination are common in such cases. Among the deaf, there is more likely to be a predominance of anxious agitation or bodily preoccupations, even to delusional extents.

As noted earlier, deafness is often caused by agents that have other sequelae as well. Retinitis pigmentosa, for example, is a genetically mediated illness in which deafness may be accompanied by blindness and mental retardation, both to varying extents. Brain damage, with or without mental retardation and other physical anomalies, may also result from maternal rubella. To the extent that such features are present, life stresses are further increased for the individual, and the diagnosis of mental illness, when it occurs, is made still more difficult.

Well-aimed treatment naturally depends on correct evaluation and diagnosis. Given the complications of deafness, a team approach is often necessary. The counselor should contribute by being able to recognize and gauge, to some extent, when something is wrong. To do so, he should know manual language well; he should also have sufficient knowledge of or have spent enough time with normal deaf people to be able to distinguish qualities of thought and attitude that are normal variations indigenous to deaf subculture and its general shared experience from qualities that are deviant enough to represent impending illness.

Psychiatric referral should clarify the diagnostic picture, at times with the assistance of psychometric or psychological tests. Relatively specific medications are available for both schizophrenia and manic-depressive disease, and the remission rate achieved is considerable. Pharmacological and other agents can also alleviate an involutional psychosis. The psychoses especially, but often disorders in the neurotic range as well, require long-term supportive psychotherapy and close follow-up with deaf patients. The guiding rule should be that anything that can go wrong will usually do so, and close interdigitation between counselor and psychiatric agency must be maintained to intercept problems before they get out of hand.

Clear communication is a major problem for the deaf; it is one that must be overcome also between the various arms of the helping forces. Clear, open, and frequent contact is required so that goals can be revised and plans altered seriatim in accordance with the level that the patient's skills, potentials, and fluctuating state of illness allow. Minor events demand prompt intervention to prevent them from becoming fullblown crises, and often agency personnel, regardless of what their discipline may be, must run interference for the deaf and psychiatrically ill client if rehabilitation plans are to continue and succeed.

Case histories are omitted here for the sake of brevity (see Altshuler, 1964; Grinker et al., 1971; Rainer, 1966; Rainer and Altshuler, 1970; and Rainer, Altshuler, and Kallmann, 1969), but given the team approach and close follow-up, results are achievable that at least are comparable to those possible with hearing patients and clients. Indeed, in view of the pervasive effects of the handicap, such successes are both remarkable and striking. The alert and flexible counselor, thus, has a role to play which can be exciting, effective, and highly gratifying personally.

SUMMARY

This chapter reviews normal development in both deaf and hearing persons. It outlines how the impingement of deafness and other handicapping conditions at times accompanying it can give rise to characteristics that can be tentatively generalized as common for deaf psychiatric patients and clients. The range of psychiatric illness is reviewed, along with alterations in clinical form that have been found typical for the deaf. How the counselor can recognize, intercede, and help effectively is stressed.

REFERENCES

Altshuler, K. Z. 1964. Personality traits and depressive symptoms in the deaf. *In* J. Wortis (ed.), Recent Advances in Biological Psychiatry. Plenum Press, New York.

Altshuler, K. Z. 1968. Reaction to and management of sensory loss: Blindness and deafness. *In* B. Schoenberg, D. Peretz, and A. Carr (eds.), Loss and Grief. Columbia University Press, New York.

Altshuler, K. Z. 1971. Studies of the deaf: Relevance to psychiatric theory. Am. J. Psychiat. 127:11.

Greenberg, J. 1970. In This Sign. Holt, Rinehart, and Winston, Inc., New York.

Grinker, R. R., Sr., et al. 1971. Psychiatric Diagnosis, Therapy, and Research on the Psychotic Deaf. U. S. Department of Health, Education, and Welfare, Social and Rehabilitation Service, Washington, D. C.

Mindel, E., and Vernon, McC. 1971. They Grow in Silence. The Deaf Child and his Family. National Association of the Deaf, Silver Spring, Md.

Rainer, J. D. 1966. Interpretation, communication, and understanding. Deaf. Amer. 19:43.

Rainer, J. D., K. Z. Altshuler, and F. J. Kallmann. 1969. Family and Mental Health Problems in a Deaf Population. 2nd Ed. Charles C Thomas, Springfield, Ill.

Rainer, J. D., and K. Z. Altshuler. 1970. Expanded Mental Health Care for the Deaf: Rehabilitation and Prevention. New York State Psychiatric Institute, New York.

Schlesinger, H. S., and K. P. Meadow. 1971. Deafness and Mental Health: A Developmental Approach. Langley Porter Neuropsychiatric Institute, San Francisco.

AUDREY SIMMONS-MARTIN

8 | Early Intervention Programs

The natural teachers of an infant are his family, and his mother in particular. With her he receives his early experiences which shape his cognitive, emotional, social and, most importantly, his linguistic development.

Observations of parents and children have provided information about the childrearing strategies which seemingly are important in the development of a child. In language acquisition, for example, mothers have been observed talking to their infants about things the child is perceiving, as he perceives them, and with frequency and consistency. Mothers tend to employ questions, praise, feedback, and to engage in a high degree of interaction.

NEED FOR EARLY INTERVENTION

Evidence has accumulated that systematic consultations with mothers about ways of teaching their children improve the children's and their own ability. Just as all parents need to employ positive maternal child care techniques, so must the parent of a hearing-impaired child. That parent most certainly requires knowledge about the effect of parent-child interaction upon language acquisition and development. Receiving little feedback, the parent of the hearing-impaired child may extinguish the behaviors which she otherwise would naturally employ. The vast majority

125

of parents, if given an idea of the principles of language growth, do a tremendous amount for their babies.

Ideally, help should be offered while the hearing-impaired child is still an infant because the early years, even months, appear to be crucial to all development, but especially language development. By 36 months of age, a normally developing child has the ability to understand most of the basic constructs underlying his language system. Unfortunately, many parents are not equipped with a practical knowledge of this early development nor do they understand the role of audition or vision. Furthermore, they probably lack knowledge about the relation of the auditory and visual processes involved in the hearing-impaired child's language development.

Rehabilitation Needs

In order to get the family and the hearing-impaired child into the mainstream of management, aggressive action needs to be directed toward alerting the community to the handicap of deafness and more specifically to the urgency of early detection. The many publics of a community need the information, but medically based professionals have a particular need. Pediatricians, nurses, general practitioners, and well-baby clinic personnel should be made aware of the importance of the early years and especially of the value in the early months of life of amplification. If every medical person to whom the statement is made, "Doctor, something is wrong with my child," probed deeper, a higher percentage of young children would be identified and started on their way. A first step in this information campaign might be to circulate a pamphlet released through the Alexander Graham Bell Association for the Deaf, *"Doctor, Is My Baby Deaf?"*

At the present time too many parents are being misdirected and encouraged to be complacent about their child until he is at least 3 years of age. The misinformation ranges from, "He is just a slow talker," to, "Perhaps he is mentally retarded." More often the informants see no existing problem and encourage the parents just to continue to do what they have been doing.

Not without blame are other professionals who encounter the parents after a diagnosis has been made. Well meaning, but contradictory, recommendations about procedures to follow are taken as absolutes by the parents and frequently leave them in a state of confusion and frustration. Before the parent has the knowledge to solve the problem, he frequently is bombarded with value judgments of systems of communication and prematurely forced to make a selection. If each route has been zealously recommended by a professional, a parent cannot help but find himself in a dilemma. This compounds an already serious problem. Not only must the parent work through the shock of having a handicapped child but he must also deal with an information overload at a time when he needs to concentrate his energies on learning "parenting," not becoming an educator, or selecting a school, let alone worrying about his child's friends in adulthood.

The role of a habilitationist is educating the public, alerting the medical community, and assisting in identifying infants with hearing disabilities. Upon identification, it would be to the family's advantage to receive clear guidance in obtaining assistance for the child and the family. The aid should be based upon the reality of the family's daily life. Parents of a hearing-impaired child can have complex and serious problems which are further compounded in the absence of good direction. This guidance is needed at the moment they first suspect something is wrong with their child.

PROFILE OF CID PARENT-INFANT PROGRAM

The Parent-Infant Program at Central Institute for the Deaf (CID) recognizes the needs of parents of hearing-impaired children. With guidance on an individual family basis and in group settings, these needs can be met. Parents *can* gain the necessary information and acquire the skills that will be enabling tools for them. They learn to interact with their child so as to promote his cognitive and linguistic growth.

The people who extend this guidance are teachers of the deaf with backgrounds in child development and parental counseling. They work closely with audiologists who oversee the hearing aid management. All of them function in an environment where deaf children are being educated and deaf adults return frequently.

The program focuses on *parental* involvement, is based on *normal* developmental sequences, and utilizes every decibel of *residual hearing.* Amplification is given the child at the outset, and parents are taught concerning its use.

Learning the Importance of Spoken Sound

The hearing-impaired baby does not respond to amplified sound quickly. Only after training does he begin to realize that sounds have meanings. As these meanings become useful to him, he begins to respond to them. The child must *learn* to *listen* just as he learns to use his other sense modalities. Included of course is vision needed for lipreading. The child needs to learn to look at his parent's face for information that will supplement what he hears.

The parent is instructed to use every natural opportunity to speak to her child. She is shown how to add speech to every kind of situation. She is taught to speak at the child's eye level and within range of his hearing aid microphone. The content of the talk is the focus of much discussion between teacher/counselor and parent. Because the home is most often the main environment of the young child, the language of the home is the language that parents should become skilled in using.

Learning How to Interact with Language

The features of the home environment are readily perceived through the senses. These perceptual features have verbal labels associated with them. In turn, the labels assist in the storage of the language (e.g., vocabulary) and the concepts. The concepts and vocabulary that develop from the perceptions are connected to actual experiences. Through experiences which have features in common, and which are mediated with similar language, concepts develop. Through perception, language is absorbed. The child, therefore, receives data from which to induce rules. For example, "washing" is a concept which has various linguistic forms: wash hands; wash face, hair; wash someone else's face, hands, etc.; wash dishes, pots, pans, silver; wash clothes; wash the car; wash the dog; wash the windows; wash the floors, etc. The implements are soap, sponge, washcloth, mop. The features in common are water, soap, and rubbing action, but the most *important* feature they have in common is the word "*wash.*"

We hypothesize that the word "wash" experienced in a *variety* of situations can be more readily learned by the child than the word experienced even many times in only *one* situation. There are some interesting data available which confirm this hypothesis (Kol'tsova, 1962).

Familiar everyday situations are more conducive to language learning than artificial and contrived ones in which lists of words are "taught." Therefore, a homelike setting should be the parents' classroom. There, the parent-facilitator can observe the appropriateness of the language and the interaction strategies used by the parent. The Home Demonstration Center which houses the Parent-Infant Program has proved valuable in this respect. It is conducive to a friendly exchange between teacher-counselor and parent as he proceeds to wash baby, dishes, pots and pans and floors, while "practicing" the parenting role. The furnishings are "early desperation," but are comfortable and inviting. Parents can do the things they ordinarily do at home with their young child, and guidance can be given by the teacher/counselor.

Because we want to demonstrate that it is the parent who must learn from us, we purposely schedule only one session in the home each week. The individualized program for each family evolves naturally. The individualization is further dependent upon the amount of residual hearing the child has, his intellectual ability, and the relations of parent to child, as well as the abilities of the family at the time of enrollment.

The goal for each child is reliance upon spoken language as a normal means of communication, learned through auditory and visual stimulation. Through wise ongoing maternal care, the child should accelerate in cognitive ability, maturity, and curiosity and develop a sense of well being.

Meeting Parent Needs

Parents, like children, bring a wide range of individual differences to the program. Each has a unique approach to the task of establishing a warm, personal relationship with his child. But they all can benefit from knowledge of the characteristics of normal *child growth* and *development* and how these relate to their child.

Importantly, parents must be acquainted with knowledge of the *hearing* process. This includes the implications of a hearing deficit, the need for early *amplification,* and procedures for its use.

They need help in understanding the stages of normal *language growth* so that they can develop facility in stimulating them for their own child in their own home. Most importantly, they need to strengthen their interaction with their child to maximize opportunities for his total development.

Because the parents are the first pupils in this plan, consideration must be given to their needs even more than to the child's. Deafness is more than a medical diagnosis. "It is a cultural phenomenon in which social, emotional, linguistic, and intellectual patterns and problems are inextricably bound together" (Schlesinger and Meadows, 1971). It appears, therefore, that parents need emotional support, factual information, opportunities to ventilate and socialize with other parents, and directed guidance in interaction with their deaf child.

Parents need support and understanding while they experience stages of anxiety, frustration, and guilt feelings. Mothers of deaf children who were studied were found to be more controlling, more intrusive, more didactic, less flexible, and less approving or encouraging than mothers of children with normal hearing (Schlesinger and Meadows, 1971). Instead of placing the burden of child *instruction* upon the parent, the Home Demonstration Program would place its thrust on the parent becoming *comfortable* with her child. Therefore, opportunities for the parent's enjoyment of his or her child should abound.

Counseling for the parents should be both direct and one-to-one. It should also be delivered in groups where the common denominator is age of child or deafness itself. The entire family complex should be the recipient of the counseling and guidance. The goal of family participation and education is the attainment of attitudes, insights, understandings, and skills. These are the tools needed to develop confidence and competence in assuming responsibility for a stimulating family life which promotes the development of communication skills in the child. An intervention program should be based on what we can define as the strengths of a well functioning family life.

The very nature of the child's handicap dictates the fundamental philosophy regarding overall management. One requirement is to ascertain the amount of hearing impairment and to identify its presence as early as possible. Then it is possible to proceed with intensive training of residual hearing using amplification. For many children, however, the route will be multisensory, using lipreading as well.

Managing Auditory Handicap

Important to an early intervention program is close association with an audiological clinic. The Parent-Infant Program is fortunate to be part of Central Institute for the Deaf which allows for close cooperation with the Speech and Hearing Services. The intake evaluations are made in those clinics, and retesting and follow-up management with reference to hearing aid use are ongoing activities after the family is enrolled in the Parent-Infant Program.

The audiologists meet weekly with the Home Demonstration staff and maintain records with regard to hearing levels. They note the auditory sensitivity of the children, upon which volume settings for each child are recommended. The audiologists select the hearing aid which is lent to the parent and guide the final selection of the aid that the parents will purchase.

Without a doubt, if a program of intervention is not fortunate enough to have a clinic with these services, they should adopt one. Teacher-counselors need to work closely with audiologists in order that the child may receive the best possible help. Furthermore, parents need wise audiological guidance. This assistance needs to be ongoing and available whenever parents encounter special problems.

Fundamentally, parents must become "experts" on hearing problems and their own child's problem in particular. They need to know why surgery, chiropractic medicine, acupuncture, and the like cannot restore hearing capability that does not exist. Importantly, they need to know how to exploit the hearing that *does* exist to the maximum. They need to be able to interpret the audiogram and explain it themselves to grandparents and other interested relatives and neighbors.

Parents need to learn simple facts about acoustics in relation to amplification, the effects of distance from the microphone, and environmental noise, for example. They need to know how to help their child *learn to listen* to speech in noise instead of just "hanging a hearing aid on him." They need to calibrate themselves to their child's particular aid and routinely check it every day. They need to know how to spot trouble with the aid, check batteries, cord, and earmold and attend to the child's reaction to amplified sound in various situations. Parents also need to understand about binaural versus monaural listening.

Parents need to know the limitations of their child's hearing aid and they must become experts at compensating for those limitations by: (1) getting within adequate auditory range before speaking, (2) getting to the child's eye level or getting him to theirs, (3) giving the child language meaningful to him when he is listening and/or looking, and (4) reinforcing his efforts when he listens or looks and listens.

Most importantly, parents must accept the aid for the great value it offers and, by their acceptance, set the model for the child to do the same. Regrettably, some parents respond to their feelings rather than to the child's performance and reject the aid because it is a visible sign of a handicapped child. The teacher-counselor needs to understand the cause of this rejection and help the parent come to terms with his feelings rather than forcing the issue. Meanwhile, if the teacher-counselor can demonstrate the child's response to intonation and later to his name with and without amplification, she may speed parental acceptance of the aid.

Working with Family Units

Ideally the young child should remain in his own home until the age at which separation from his mother comes easily. In the Parent-Infant Program child and family make only weekly visits to the Home Demonstration Center. During that session the teacher-counselor may demonstrate what can be done with the child at home. She may discuss the activity and let the parent demonstrate or they may engage in a fruitful discussion of a topic relative to the child's growth.

Both parents are urged to attend because both have questions and concerns. Siblings are also important members of a family group and need consideration and inclusion in a family setting. Normal hearing children have feelings and attitudes about a handicapped sibling that need to be identified and redirected (Farber, 1962). Families of hearing-impaired children are first of all *families* and, thus, have feelings similar to those of any family. They have needs, hopes, desires, and wants because of their economic, social, and educational environment; in addition they develop certain attitudes because of the presence of a handicap. Hence, the unit that meets the teacher-counselor should be the family as often as parents' jobs and siblings' school allow.

Group Meetings

Group meetings are an efficient means of transmitting general information to several family groups at once. Because there is a core of such information that parents of hearing-impaired children need, these meetings are held regularly in Central Institute for the Deaf's Parent-Infant Program. They tend to be informal in nature, but the topics range from appropriate toys to hearing aid specifications. More opportunities for parents to ventilate their feelings exist in the group meetings than in the settings with just the professional person and a single family.

Nursery Classes

As the child matures and is ready for group education, he is placed in a part-time nursery class. Parents participate in the class as well. Not only do they observe, but they also work with the children as in a cooperative nursery setting.

As parents see their own child in relation to the growth of other children, they perceive him more objectively. By observing other parents contriving and creating situations for language stimulation, they also grow in appreciation of the task. Being put in the role of a class teacher helps the parents appraise the task of school and aids them in setting realistic expectations for their child in full-time school.

In the nursery class, the learning experiences and activities are designed to satisfy the children's urge to invent, discover, construct, and create. Importantly, parents and children learn together.

STRATEGIES OF INTERVENTION

The intervention curriculum is a process whereby the teacher-counselor attempts to modify the naturally occurring dynamics within the hearing-impaired child's family for the child's benefit. In the course of the process, parents are taught about the development and acquisition of aural/oral language.

In the individual family sessions the parent is given an assignment to apply a principle or rule to a common daily situation which involves interaction between the parent and the child. Activities to promote this interaction may range from playing with a toy to setting the table, dusting, washing dishes, or any other household or yard chore. It may include picnics or trips to the grocery store or zoo.

Teacher-Counselor Strategies

The teacher-counselor may be willing and eager to initiate educational techniques, but the parent may still be coping with the shock of the diagnostic findings. Furthermore, the teacher may also be dealing with parents who do not easily learn from verbal instructions. The teacher in the parent-centered phase of the program must adjust her strategies to the parents' needs. She may at any one time be: a *reinforcer* because she supports everything positive that the mother does; an *activity director,* giving ideas to the parent who is unsure of what to do; a *modeler,* demonstrating activities appropriate for the parent to perform; and an *information seeker and giver,* sharing information about the child's physical growth, social growth, language growth, hearing loss, hearing aids, educational systems, acupuncture, and any other topic remotely or directly related to handicaps and deafness in particular.

Any single intervention session often contains many teaching strategies. Nineteen were identified by Nardine (1974). They included language expansion, language imitation, language repetition directed to the child, interpreting the child's efforts to the mother, strategy clarification, and categorization of objects and actions, to name a few. Needless to say, the roles of lipreading and amplification need frequent and meaningful interpretation to the parent who is providing the input.

Parent Strategies

Parents are encouraged to apply principles they have learned at previous sessions, at parents' meetings, or from their readings. These strategies include: (1) how to use amplification, (2) when to talk, (3) what to talk about, (4) how to talk at child's receptive language level, (5) how to use repetition, (6) how to reinforce the child's talk.

Parents of hearing-impaired children need to be familiar with the effects of limited audition and to learn strategies to compensate. Information about amplification and its use, facility in reaching the child's eye level, and speaking at a rate and within sentence boundaries that his eyes and ears can attend to are a few of the particular skills that parents of the hearing impaired need to learn.

The language *stimulation* can vary both in quality and quantity. The quality should be appropriate to the child's language comprehension age. While quantity is important, the kind of input is even more crucial. Just "talk, talk, talk" is inappropriate, but rather the input should match the child's thought at the moment it occurs. This match should take place frequently and meaningfully. Since no one knows enough about what any particular child is thinking at any given moment, the curriculum cannot be planned. It is hoped that parents can generalize the strategy through clear examples and guided self-evaluation.

In order to help the child see what is relevant in the verbal barrage, the parent needs to learn to talk about the things *the child* is interested in, *his* toys, *his* clothing, *his* food. Since he is very much in the "here and now" stage, the objects should be present and available for the child to handle and explore as they are being talked about. Frequently parents complain about this strategy. It is as if they are talking to themselves, but, through storage over time, the child can develop a language system for his later use (Simmons-Martin, 1971).

The kind of language mothers use with their young children has been analyzed. The sentences mothers tend to use with their young hearing children were short and grammatically complete (Broen, 1972; Brown and Bellugi, 1964). The sentences were also clearly defined in the mother's speech by pauses marking the boundaries. Others have shown that speech addressed to young children was syntactically less complex (Philip, 1973; Snow, 1972). Imperative and declarative forms were most often used. Except for story-telling situations, the rate was slower for younger children. Mother's speech to infants had a smaller range of vocabulary than that with older children and was more redundant. They often repeated what they had said with and without variations, but they rarely used meaningless repetitions or produced broken sentences. Expansion of utterances is a strategy most parents use early in their language teaching, but modeling seems to be of value later in the acquisition process (Cazden, 1972).

A family's daily routine builds in much repetition. It is easy to see that the same foods, the same activities, the same clothing get labeled frequently in the course of a day. Through frequent exposure the child can move from the awareness stage of language learning to the absorption level. Such repetition as the home provides is essential for early learning (Simmons, 1966).

The language style of the parent is the element of importance. That is, the child's *creative concepts* must be matched with language rather than ignored or rejected. It is still an open question whether reinforcement or feedback is important to language development or whether rich stimulation or exposure is sufficient. In *parent* education, however, it is the *parents* who need reinforcement. The infant may not be reinforcing the mother with coos, laughs, babbles, and in other ways as hearing children do. Therefore, praise and positive support should definitely be a responsibility of the person shaping mother's behavior. At the same time parents must be guided to give reinforcement themselves to the child's efforts.

Because parents are individuals with a wide range of needs, each is helped to perfect his or her own style or strategy. Some parents are given models to imitate, some are given specific instruction, some are given *Chats with Johnny's Parents* (Simmons-Martin, 1975) to follow and discuss. For all parents, videotaping of their individual sessions has proved beneficial. In viewing their tape, the parents become aware of their own abilities to communicate with their child and areas in which they must correct their procedures. Self-correction is more effective than criticism from the teacher.

Curriculum in Summary

An intervention program should be developmental rather than remedial. Because each child is unique and each family make-up differs, the actual content of instruction will vary greatly. Possibly it would be useful to list what may be common threads for the children's development:

1. Parents need to become effective educational agents with their own children by being *good parents,* not second rate teachers.
2. They need assistance in understanding hearing and the implications of a hearing loss and how to interpret their child's loss to others.
3. They need to know how to exploit the child's hearing to the maximum. Therefore, they need simple facts about acoustics in relation to hearing aids, environmental noise, distance from microphone, and binaural versus monaural listening.
4. They need to know about linguistic development in children and provide the models for their child's growth.
5. Parents need to be guided in assisting their child to comprehend language and in employing simple reinforcement procedures.
6. They need an understanding of lipreading and how to "stage set" their own environment for the best possible viewing by the child.
7. They need to know children in general, how they play and grow and respond to healthy measures of loving care and purposeful discipline.

Certainly, a home demonstration program is not a panacea for the problems of parents of hearing-impaired children. However, it does enable a parent to become more effective by providing meaningful experiences which provide the basis for his cognitive, emotional, social, and, most importantly, his linguistic development.

REFERENCES

Broen, P. A. Dec. 1972. The verbal environment of the language learning child. ASHA Monogr. #17. Washington, D. C.
Brown, R. W., and U. Bellugi. 1964. Three processes in the child's acquisition of syntax. Harvard Ed. Rev. 34:133–151.

Cazden, C. B. 1972. *Child Language and Education*, Holt, Rinehart & Winston, Inc., New York.

Farber, B. 1962. Effects of severely mentally retarded child on the family. *In* Trapp and Hemelstein (eds.), Readings on the Exceptional Child, pp. 227–246. Appleton-Century-Crofts, Inc., New York.

Kol'tsova, N. M. 1962. The formation of higher nervous activity of the child. Psychol. Rev. 69:344–354.

Nardine, F. 1974. Parents as a teaching resource. Volta Rev. March: 172–177.

Philip, J. R. 1973. Syntax and vocabulary of mother's speech to young children: age and sex comparison. Child Dev. 44:182–185.

Schlesinger, H. S., and K. P. Meadows. 1971. Deafness and Mental Health: A Developmental Approach. Langley Porter Neuropsychiatric Institute, San Francisco.

Simmons, A. A. 1966. Language growth for the pre-nursery deaf child. Volta Rev. 68:3.

Simmons-Martin, A. 1971. Relationships to language and hearing. *In* L. E. Connor (ed.), Speech for the Deaf. Alexander Graham Bell Association, Washington, D. C.

Simmons-Martin, A. 1975. *Chats with Johnny's Parents.* Alexander Graham Bell Association, Washington, D. C.

Snow, C. E. 1972. Mother's speech to children learning language. Child Dev. 43:549–565.

Rehabilitation Programs

⑨

BRIAN BOLTON

The goal of rehabilitation is the preparation of the deaf client for independent living in our vastly complex society. His/her satisfaction with life will
be greatest if he/she is participating in a variety of social and cultural
activities and making a recognized contribution to the maintenance of
societal functioning. Therefore, rehabilitation services must be dedicated
to the preparation of the "whole client." Work can be viewed as the
central theme around which life in contemporary societies is organized;
thus, vocational adjustment may reasonably be taken as the ultimate goal
of rehabilitation programming. The many specialized supporting services
which are required to ameliorate the personal-social deficits of deaf rehabilitation clients can be viewed as building blocks in a preparatory
sequence which, hopefully, result in successful vocational adjustment.

Rehabilitation of deaf clients is not fundamentally different than
rehabilitation of blind clients, psychiatric patients, or any other group.
The basic philosophy and services are the same. However, each disability
group has special problems and unique needs. The basic rehabilitation
techniques must be adapted to these unique needs. This chapter consists of
three sections: (1) brief descriptions of the specialized rehabilitation
procedures required by deaf clients, (2) capsule summaries of five major
research and demonstration projects which were designed to serve severely
disabled deaf clients, and (3) a list of some two dozen principles of service
and policy implications which were derived from the available literature on
rehabilitation of deaf clients.

137

REHABILITATION SERVICE COMPONENTS

This section presents an overview of the various rehabilitation services required to prepare deaf clients for satisfactory independent living. Every client will require a different combination of services, each tailored to his/her unique needs. A relatively long program (2 years or more) can be anticipated for the most underdeveloped clients; others will attain adequate to superior levels of competence in 6 months or less. Rehabilitation programming for deaf clients must be flexible. Psychological assessment is a continuous process which does not cease when the initial rehabilitation plan is formulated; rehabilitation services must be modified to best help the client as he/she changes during the process. While the service components are described separately for the purpose of clarity of presentation, it should be understood that, in practice, the various service elements are integrated into a cohesive operational program. The various rehabilitation services can be placed in three categories: (1) case management and counseling, (2) personal-social preparatory services, and (3) vocational preparatory services. Within each of these broad categories are included several specific program components which are discussed as follows.

Case Management and Counseling

The case manager occupies a central role in the administration of the rehabilitation program in that he/she: (1) coordinates the various service components, and (2) provides counseling and guidance for the client on a continuous schedule. Program coordination for deaf clients is similar to the coordination of programs for clients with other disabilities; the counseling process is usually different.

Deaf clients generally experience the same kinds of problems and difficulties that hearing clients do, although deafness does present some unique situations. Therefore, the basic nature of the counseling process is unchanged, but the mode of interaction is different. The critical aspect is, of course, the fidelity of communication between counselor and client. The typical client will have difficulty in expressing his/her concerns or problems; thus, the counselor will have difficulty understanding the client and communicating that understanding to the client. The counselor must be especially alert to nonverbal aspects of communication. Often the affective component of the interaction will be entirely nonverbal because the client will not possess the means to "intellectualize" his/her feelings. As a general rule, the counselor should concentrate on specifics (incidents, persons, etc.) and avoid talking about "things in general." Counseling with deaf clients often reduces to rather directive "guidance" in the context of information giving. This is a necessary aspect of the total counseling process with deaf clients and should not be viewed as evidence of failure in counseling. Stewart (1971) has written an excellent discussion of the issues and problems in counseling deaf clients which is illustrated with case excerpts; the following points have been abstracted from his presentation:

1. The nature and principles of the counseling relationship with deaf clients are no different than those that characterize counseling with nondeaf clients; rather, it is the implementation which differs.
2. Because of the language limitations of most deaf clients, the counselor must adopt a manner of expression comparable to the client's and employ a focused questioning approach to encourage the client to elaborate on his/her thoughts and feelings.
3. Client understanding will be enhanced when the counselor asks briefer and more specific questions; thus, open-end, unstructured questions are minimized in favor of a structuring orientation.
4. Information giving is basic to effective counseling since many deaf clients lack necessary information which makes successful counseling possible; thus, the counselor must be prepared to use a variety of guidance materials with deaf clients.
5. The counselor will often have to go outside the counseling relationship per se and provide assistance with the client's daily activities, especially those that will increase his/her knowledge and skills in relating to people.
6. The counselor must be aware of societal conditions and situations which present barriers to deaf persons and which are almost impossible to change, and help the deaf client to understand and accept his/her limitations.

The goal of counseling is to prepare the deaf client to become an independent, mature decision-maker, able to deal competently with everyday problems. In order to achieve this goal, the client must have an accurate understanding of the function and purpose of the rehabilitation program and his/her responsibilities and obligations and he/she must make a personal commitment to the goal of the program. This requires a thorough orientation by the counselor and other rehabilitation personnel. After the client is oriented to the rehabilitation program (a process which may require 2 weeks or longer), the case manager should periodically convene case conferences with all personnel in attendance for the purpose of assessing progress and modifying the rehabilitation plan as needed.

Personal-Social Preparatory Services

Comprehensive personal-social adjustment services constitute the foundation of the rehabilitation program for most deaf clients. Minimal competence in all areas of personal-social functioning must be attained before independent living is a realistic goal. Four service components are outlined in this section: supervised living, personal adjustment training, recreational and cultural activities, and group counseling.

Supervised Living While most comprehensive rehabilitation facilities have provisions for residential housing, the majority of rehabilitation projects serving deaf clients do not. Living arrangements can be made for clients in private homes (usually on a contract basis), the YMCA or YWCA, or apartments. Deaf young adults housed in apartments will require intensive supervision and assistance initially. Ideally, clients are first placed in private homes or the "Y" and later "graduated" to trial independent living situations. This shift should be coordinated with the client's progress in the personal adjustment training curriculum. Deaf clients will mature most rapidly if classroom-type instruction is paralleled by opportunities to apply skills in realistic situations in the surrounding community. An independent living program is described in detail by Rice and Milligan (1973).

Personal Adjustment Training Personal adjustment training (PAT) refers to the acquisition of information and basic skills related to satisfactory personal-social functioning. A set of topics, with examples of teaching units, which comprise a PAT program is outlined in Table 1. The two primary methods of instruction employed are individual tutoring and small group "lectures." Individual study and group work may be used as supplementary procedures. Visual aids in the form of charts, slides, manuals, and captioned films are important teaching media for the PAT instructor. A large number of captioned films with accompanying lesson guides is available through several regional media centers for the deaf. The interested reader should contact the Media Services and Captioned Films division of the Bureau of Education for the Handicapped for more information. The enterprising PAT instructor can construct a variety of charts and visual displays to enhance the learning process. Workbooks and practice exercises greatly improve the acquisition and retention of basic educational skills. Many commercially available teaching/learning aids can be adapted for the purposes of developing personal-social skills in deaf clients.

Recreational Activities Approximately one-half of modern man's waking hours are spent in nonwork activities. Thus, the constructive use of leisure time is a topic of some importance. Most people develop avocational interests or hobbies, usually in an area dissimilar from their occupations. Avocational interests, like their vocational counterpart, require opportunities and experience to flourish. Thus, many deaf clients do not have well developed avocational interests or varied leisure activities.

Table 1. Personal adjustment training areas of preparation

Areas	Examples
Communication skills	Manual Sign language, fingerspelling, vocabulary development, writing, and reading
Basic educational skills	Arithmetic, measurements (time, temperature, weight, etc.), map and graph reading
Personal hygiene	Grooming, etiquette, cleanliness, medical care, mental health
Marriage and family	Sex and reproduction, legal aspects, courtship, responsibilities
Citizenship	Voting, driving, police, government, social security, law
Leisure	Social organizations, clubs, church, hobbies, recreation
Independent living skills	Leases and contracts, housekeeping, nutrition, laundry, budgeting, safety, taxes
Consumer services	Purchasing, credit buying, interest and charges, banking, insurance
Community services	Post office, transportation

A comprehensive recreational program has two major goals: (1) the development of a variety of leisure-time pursuits through a planned program of activities, and (2) the expansion of cultural horizons through exposure to places and events of historical and artistic significance. The former is accomplished by participation in games (cards, bowling, team sports, etc.), membership in clubs (photography, wildlife, boating, etc.), and solitary activities (collections, craftwork, reading, etc.). Cultural interests can be stimulated through captioned films and visits to museums, art galleries, historical sites, and various industries. Recreational activities also serve as a vehicle for training and experience in social interaction with peers, staff, and members of the community.

Group Counseling The social immaturity of deaf young adults is nowhere more evident than in group discussion situations. The interaction that is observed is often comparable to the preadolescent behavior of hearing youth. Thus, group counseling is not really "counseling" at all, but rather a technique for learning group skills, e.g., listening to other people, discussing controversial topics, respecting differing points of view, etc. Group sessions should focus on problem-sharing as much as possible because deaf clients tend to experience many of the same types of difficulties in their rehabilitation programs: awareness that one's problems are not entirely unique is comforting and provides a basis for discussion.

Limited communication skills make the optimal group size six to eight clients.

Vocational Preparatory Services

The goal of vocational services is to prepare the client for placement on a job in which he can function sufficiently well to support himself. Vocational preparation entails much more than the acquisition of skills; the role of a worker must be learned. Most adolescents begin by mowing lawns, washing dishes, delivering newspapers, babysitting, etc., and gradually develop the responsible attitudes and behaviors that constitute vocational maturity. Deaf youth who are deprived of the requisite developmental experiences cannot simply be taught a trade and placed in a job. Vocational maturity in deaf clients can be fostered through a sequence of four services: vocational evaluation, vocational adjustment, skill training, and job placement.

Vocational Evaluation The process of vocational evaluation is conducted in the standard workshop setting. It is oriented around two major concerns: (1) the evaluation of work behavior, including attitudes, values, and habits, and (2) the assessment of training capacity. The first purpose, then, is to construct a diagnostic profile of the client's "work personality" which will form the basis for the vocational adjustment phase. The second purpose is to develop a training potential profile to assist the counselor and client in selecting an appropriate skill training area. The vocational evaluation process actually begins with the personality assessment which takes place during the comprehensive psychological evaluation. The client's "work personality" is just an extension of his total functioning personality; thus, the assessment of vocational maturity is distinguished by the attention paid to specific behaviors essential to successful vocational adjustment. Most workshops use a work behavior evaluation form which is completed periodically to record problem areas (the diagnostic profile) and assess progress during vocational adjustment.

Vocational Adjustment Most deaf clients require an extended period of work adjustment in order to acquire the attitudes and habits associated with the role of reliable worker. The vocational adjustment process applied to deaf clients involves the same behavior shaping techniques that are effective with hearing clients. The essential characteristics of the adjustment process are: a work environment which is similar to actual employment conditions, the use of incentives and rewards to modify behavior, an emphasis on work attitudes as well as habits, and understanding, yet firm, supervision by experienced counselor-foremen. The work adjustment phase begins with the client's diagnostic profile assembled during the vocational evaluation. Specific deficits and problem areas receive special attention and serve to introduce the client to the learning process. Periodic assessments provide objective measures of progress and signal the client's readiness for vocational skill training. The counselor should anticipate a lengthy work adjustment for most clients and not be disappointed at relatively slow progress, especially early in the program.

Skill Training Many deaf clients come to rehabilitation facilities with some vocational training experience, especially those clients from state residential schools. Their preparation is often inadequate, but it may provide a foundation for skill training in some areas. Regardless of the client's previous experience or lack of it, selection of a training area should not be made for the client based on administrative considerations. Counselor and client together should explore the vocational possibilities, considering the client's training potential profile, the results of psychological tests, and the client's expressed interests. The temptation to assign clients to traditional deaf occupations (printing, shoe repair, etc.) or unskilled areas (laundry, custodial, etc.) should be strenuously resisted. Deaf persons are often undertrained and subsequently underemployed because the special arrangements that may be required for placement in appropriate training areas are not made.

Counselors should recognize, and explain to their deaf clients, that vocational training will generally take longer for deaf than hearing clients (about half again as long on the average). This is not because deaf clients are "slow learners," but reflects the influence of impaired communication on the instructional process. Repeated demonstrations are often necessary. Thus, the vocational instructor who is training deaf clients should have smaller classes. Regardless of the training area, vocational tutoring will probably be a necessary adjunct service. Only through the provision of intensive vocational training can the underemployment of deaf persons, as evidenced by their concentration in semiskilled and unskilled occupations, be reduced.

Job Placement The job placement service consists of four phases. First, rehabilitation workers must educate potential employers regarding deafness. Job finding is a continuous activity which aims to expand the job market for deaf trainees. Second, the client must be prepared to present himself positively to the potential employer, e.g., he should be coached in completing an application form, handling himself in the interview, dressing and grooming appropriately, etc. Third, the actual placement of the client on the job may entail helping with orientation and locating suitable living arrangements. Fourth, deaf clients often need continuing assistance in adjusting to their new situations. The counselor should contact the employer on a regular basis and be available in case of any "emergencies." While placement is the immediate goal of rehabilitation, long-term adjustment is the ultimate responsibility. An on-going follow-up program is the best insurance against unsuccessful outcomes.

RESULTS OF REHABILITATION PROGRAMS

During the past decade several research and demonstration projects have been conducted in existing rehabilitation facilities for the purpose of serving severely handicapped deaf clients. Clients were drawn from the populations of deaf youth who were unsuccessful in school and chronically maladjusted deaf adults. Five large-scale innovative programs are summarized in this section.

Boston Project

Lawrence and Vescovi (1967) reported an exploratory service program conducted at Morgan Memorial, Inc. from 1965–1967. One hundred twenty-six deaf clients from six New England states were served in a vocational evaluation and work adjustment center. Major services provided were: vocational and psychological evaluation, work adjustment, rehabilitation counseling, social casework, tutoring and personal adjustment training, and a summer enrichment program for students. Most of the sample (80%) was designated multiply handicapped, a majority were male (69%), half (52%) were between 15 and 24 years of age, and half were considered to be functionally illiterate (47%). Sixty percent of the project clients were judged to have received positive benefits from their programs (e.g., they were employed or enrolled in academic or vocational training courses). Forty percent achieved full-time employment. Communication difficulties constituted the greatest problem for clients; it is imperative that staff responsible for deaf clients be fluent in manual language. The authors concluded that deaf clients can be successfully served in rehabilitation facilities by employing a special core staff of professionals.

Hot Springs Project (I)

Blake (1970) described the first deaf project carried out at the Hot Springs Rehabilitation Center. The purpose of the project was to assess the feasibility of providing services to deaf clients in a comprehensive rehabilitation center with a special staff. Client services were offered in medical, psychological, social, and vocational areas. The project sample of 131 clients from the southwest states included the more difficult clients in the referring counselors' caseloads. The majority were young (90% between 16 and 25 years), male (70%), white (80%), and single (only six were married or had ever been married). They were slightly below average on the WAIS Performance Scale (mean of 95) and possessed academic skills equivalent to those of the average fourth grader. Considering the "difficulty" of the clients, the results of the project were excellent. Fifty-five percent of the clients completed vocational training courses and received graduation certificates (at an average cost of $2,400 for an average program length of 8 months). However, 38% dropped out or were discharged. At 6 months follow-up, 41% of all clients were employed full-time. Those clients who graduated from training courses were more successful: 61% were employed full-time, and only 10% had not worked or continued their education. It was estimated that 85% of the clients evidenced improvements in some area of functioning. Two conclusions of this project deserve emphasis: (1) deaf clients require extended periods of personal, social, and work adjustment before admission to formal vocational training programs, and (2) enhancement of the communication skills of both deaf clients and professional staff is essential to the provision of effective rehabilitation services.

St. Louis Project

Hurwitz (1971) described a 5-year project conducted at the St. Louis Jewish Vocational Service to serve deaf young adults. The program emphasized vocational and social rehabilitation; the major vehicle of service was the prevocational adjustment workshop. Other components of the work preparedness program were evaluation, on-the-job training, skill training, and job placement. Clients were prepared for and assisted with arrangements for independent community living. The majority of the 265 clients served were between 16 and 20 years of age (66%) and few were married (12%). The average IQ was 92 (21% were below 80) and the average reading achievement level was 3.5 grades (8% were above sixth grade). Approximately one-half of the clients could be considered to be multiply handicapped on the basis of diagnosed physical or neuropsychological conditions alone. Results were as follows: one-half of the clients were placed in competitive employment (mostly in semiskilled or unskilled jobs), 7% in sheltered workshops, and 19% were recommended for advanced training. At follow-up, 64% of a random sample of clients were employed. The most impressive statistic reported was: 86% of the clients were financially dependent at referral, and 76% were self-sufficient at follow-up.

Chicago Project

The deaf project conducted by the Chicago Jewish Vocational Service terminated in 1972 after 5 years of research and services to deaf clients (Chicago Jewish Vocational Service, 1974). The unifying theme of the service program was vocational development; major services provided were: vocational evaluation, work adjustment training, counseling and placement, tutoring in communication and basic skills, family counseling, and an information and referral service. The project served a total of 710 deaf clients, 457 of whom received substantial vocational services. A "core" sample of 309 clients who completed the psychological testing battery possessed the following characteristics: 52% male, median age of 22 years, 55% white, 68% single, 23% self-supporting, mean IQ of 99 on the Revised Beta, and manual communication skills were rated average. A follow-up study ascertained that one-half (49%) of the clients who received substantial services were employed (two-thirds had held a job) and 22% were placed in various training and preparatory programs. The project sponsored several supplementary programs, e.g., coaching classes for the civil service examination for post office employment, a summer enrichment program and work study program for deaf youth, and extensive community organizations, including a monthly calendar of events and a directory of services.

Hot Springs Project (II)

The second Hot Springs Project, which was designed to provide comprehensive services to the most severely handicapped deaf clients, is summarized by Bolton (1974). A total of 235 clients received extensive psychological evaluations, counseling and guidance, personal-social preparatory services, and vocational adjustment and training during the 5-year project. The "multiply handicapped" syndrome is evident from the sample description: two-thirds were male (70%), most were young (78% aged 25 years or younger), almost all were single (97%), two-thirds were white (69%), most were supported by their families (84%), one-half (49%) received a high school diploma or certificate, one-half (56%) had previous work experience, manual communication skills were rated fair, and the median WAIS IQ was 91. A series of three annual follow-up surveys documented the success of the project: one-half of the clients were employed in the competitive labor market at an average salary of 75 dollars per week in semiskilled and unskilled occupations. Of those clients who completed their training programs (52%), two-thirds were employed competitively. A regression analysis isolated the two major predictors of employment: previous work experience and completion of a vocational training program.

PRINCIPLES OF REHABILITATION SERVICE

It can be concluded from the results of the five demonstration service projects that at least one-half of severely handicapped deaf young adults can be rehabilitated (more properly, habilitated) with a core program of vocational and social services. Poor communication skills constitute the single most critical barrier to effective rehabilitation services and subsequent vocational and community adjustment.

The following guidelines or *implications for practice* were derived, in part, from the final reports of the service demonstration studies discussed above:

1. The ability to communicate in manual Sign language is prerequisite to serving deaf clients; manual sign language is not "signed English," but a separate visual-graphic communication system which constitutes a native language to many deaf persons.

2. Deaf persons possess the same intellectual capacity as hearing persons, including the ability to solve "abstract" problems; however, they are deficient in their mastery of the common symbol system we know as language.

3. Many deaf persons exhibit retarded personal-social development as a result of experiential deprivation; there is no evidence to support the notion of a "deaf personality."

4. Counseling with deaf clients must be situation specific; language difficulties prevent the meaningful discussion of "philosophical" issues. Information giving is an important dimension of the counseling process.

5. Deaf clients require thorough evaluation as a basis for rehabilitation planning; essential aspects are: case history review, psychological testing, situational assessment, and vocational evaluation.

6. The client should be involved in the planning of his rehabilitation program; only through understanding can commitment develop. Giving the deaf client responsibility is the first step toward independence.

7. The rehabilitation program should be as realistic as possible to maximize the transfer of learning. Practical experiences such as independent living training and trial job placements should be utilized whenever possible; the community can be used as a "field test" area.

8. Deaf clients will generally require a longer period of time to complete most services and reach a specified level of competence than hearing clients. Rehabilitation programming should take this into account rather than foster unrealistic expectations in deaf clients.

9. Psychological assessment and vocational evaluation should focus on the qualitative aspects of performance (how the client approached the task, his characteristic behaviors, etc.) as well as the quantitative aspects.

10. Deaf clients require thorough orientation to all activities; directions must be simplified and should include demonstrations whenever possible.

11. Personal-social preparatory services (PAT training, group counseling, living arrangements, etc.) are the cornerstone of the rehabilitation program for deaf clients; one-half of the total program may be devoted to personal-social preparation in some cases.

12. Most deaf clients will require an extended period of work adjustment before skill training can be initiated.

13. Deaf clients require more intensive instructional supervision in vocational training programs; thus, lower staff-student ratios should be arranged.

14. Deaf clients should receive special vocational tutoring in conjunction with their vocational training programs.

15. Deaf clients often require various supportive services such as interpreting, letter writing, explanation of rules, etc.

16. Employer education and continued contact after placement can greatly improve the deaf client's probability of successful vocational adjustment. On-the-job "counseling" should be available on short notice to deal with any problems that may arise.

17. The success of the deaf client's rehabilitation can be enhanced by involving his family in the program whenever possible. Their support and interest may have special meaning for the client.

The following *policy implications* were prepared by the author at the request of Rehabilitation Services Administration (RSA) officials:

1. Severely handicapped deaf clients can be prepared for successful vocational adjustment and independent community living by rehabilitation programs which provide special services for them; rehabilitation programs designed to meet the unique needs of deaf clients should be developed in all federally funded facilities.

2. Successful rehabilitation of severely handicapped deaf clients does not conclude with completion of training or job placement, but, rather, is a continuing process which extends into the community; support services should be provided to ex-clients through counseling and referral agencies and coordinated with the rehabilitation programs.

3. Rehabilitation programming for many severely handicapped deaf youth begins at school termination; rehabilitation services should be initiated before termination and reflect a cooperative working arrangement between the two institutions.

4. The tremendous retardation in language development and academic achievement which characterizes severely handicapped deaf youth cannot be significantly ameliorated by remedial services; all deaf children should be enrolled in special preschool classes at age 2 and their parents should

receive training from educational specialists in order to prevent the "multiply handicapped" syndrome.

5. Severely handicapped deaf clients require more intensive services over a longer period of time than the average client; financial appropriations for rehabilitation services should reflect this higher cost per client.

6. Severely handicapped deaf clients possess average intelligence and perform within the average range on ability and aptitude tests which tap "native" capacities; expanded psychometric research programs to investigate the ability requirements of occupations outside the stereotyped deaf areas should be funded.

7. Counselors need special training in order to effectively serve severely handicapped deaf clients; stipends should be available to students and counselors who express an interest in working with deaf clients.

8. Because they usually possess excellent communication skills and an intimate knowledge of the deaf community, deaf persons and hearing persons with deaf parents should be the focus of recruiting efforts by university rehabilitation counselor training programs.

REFERENCES

Blake, G. 1970. An experiment in serving deaf adults in a comprehensive rehabilitation center. Final Report, SRS Grant No. RD-1932-S, Arkansas Rehabilitation Service, Little Rock, Ark.

Bolton, B. 1974. A behavior-oriented treatment program for deaf clients in a comprehensive rehabilitation center. Amer. J. Orthopsychiatry 44: 376–385.

Chicago, Jewish Vocational Service. 1974. The Chicago project for the deaf. Final Report, SRS Grant No. RD-1576. Chicago Jewish Vocational Service, Chicago.

Hurwitz, S. 1971. Habilitation of deaf young adults. Final Report, SRS Grant No. RD-1804-S, Jewish Employment and Vocational Service, St. Louis.

Lawrence, C. A., and G. M. Vescovi. 1967. Deaf adults in New England: An exploratory service program. Final Report, SRS Grant No. RD-1576, Morgan Memorial, Inc., Boston.

Rice, B. D., and T. Milligan. 1973. A structured approach to independent living training for young multiply handicapped deaf adults. J. Rehabil. Deaf 6 (4):38–43.

Stewart, L. 1971. The nature of counseling with deaf people. In A. Sussman and L. Stewart (eds.), Counseling with Deaf People, pp. 55–86. Deafness Research and Training Center, New York.

Index